Intentive Touch

The Cohen Method of Soft Tissue Therapy

Jeff Cohen

Table of Contents

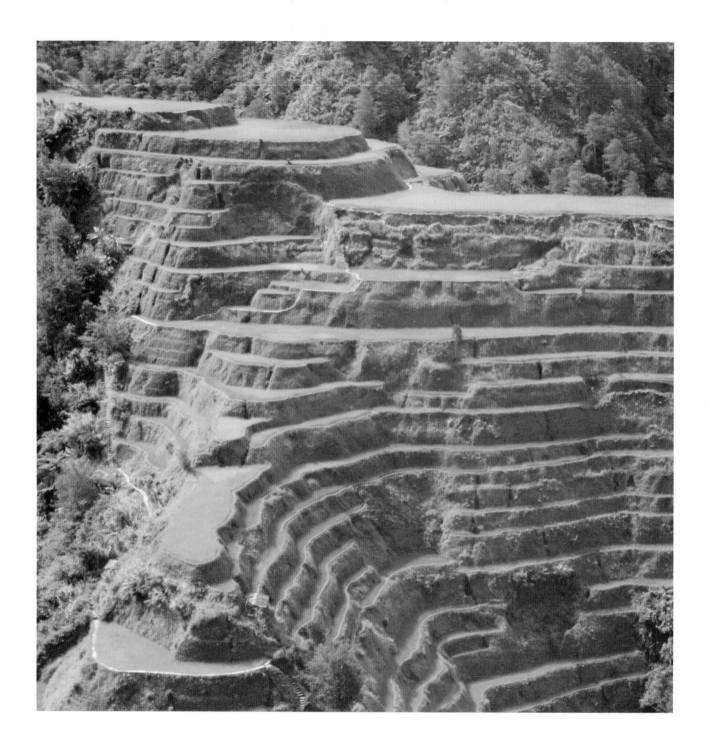

Forward

For years I have been asked to share the method and technique that I use in my practice. I have been hesitant, as I was taught in a one-on-one teacher-apprentice format. It has been a challenge to translate that experience into a western format. The following book is designed to give a sense of the feelings and connections that bind the practitioner and the subject, which are crucial to the methods I learned.

I did the majority of my training in the Philippines from 1979-1985 with a healer from the Bontoc Mountain Province named Ina Facucad Fanged. My brother Gordon had suffered a spinal cord injury from a car accident, which is what spearheaded this healing journey. As she worked on Gordon, Facucad began to teach me her healing technique, called Hilot. Her knowledge was extensive, and she generously shared many insights with me. We had a unique relationship that transcended language, as neither of us spoke the other's, except for a few words and expressions. There were many gaps and disconnects between our two cultures. At times I was not sure how I should interpret and apply the unspoken concepts, but this did not stop the transfer of knowledge; it just forced me to expand my capacity to embrace the universal concepts of love, compassion, and healing.

Subsequently I trained with other master healers in the Philippines, who also shared some of their healing traditions with me. As an outsider, I was blessed to be trusted with some of the oral traditions of these masters. I later augmented this knowledge and experience with explorations into relevant concepts and practices in western medicine. The result is a unique fusion of traditional wisdom and cutting-edge research. Just as my teachers and mentors, both in the Philippines and in the U.S., were willing to share their knowledge with me, this book is my way of offering my insights to you.

Though Hilot exists throughout the Philippine archipelago, it is not standardized. The majority of my apprenticeships took place while I watched the different Hilot masters working on problems arising from Gordon's paraplegia. As different as each technique was, each proved to have definite positive effects. It was fascinating to see different approaches create similar results.

Each of my teachers had a unique method, yet there were certain fundamental principles common to them all. What is most important for me in sharing my insights is to extend the community feeling and function that is woven into the spirit of helping people relieve their pain. Being in the Philippines opened me up to see and feel, and therefore know that there are multiple layers of understanding and many ways to express fundamental things. While in Bontoc, I experienced firsthand the slow pace of tribal village living. I could not help but observe and absorb the elements of a different approach to appreciating the interconnectedness and pulse of life that runs through all things.

Through my journey, I have developed Intentive Touch: The Cohen Method of Soft Tissue Therapy.

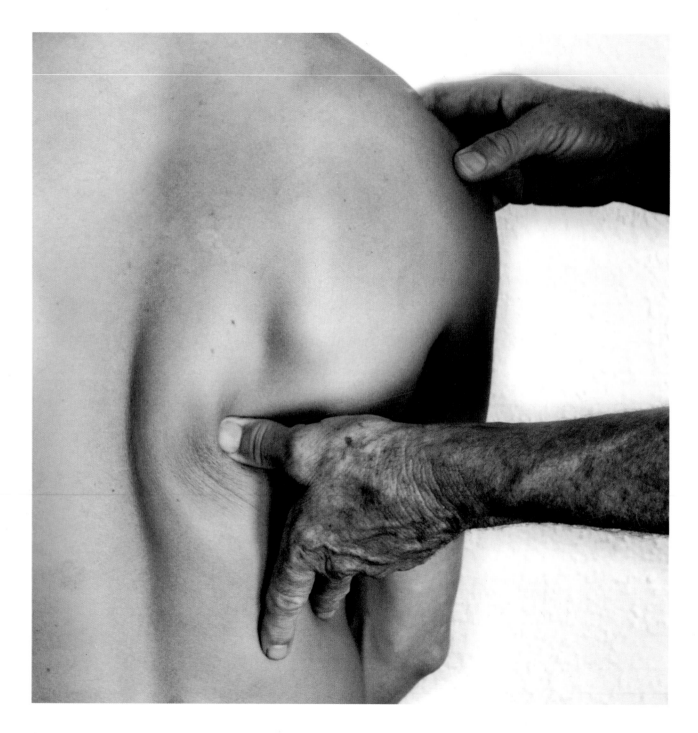

Intentive Touch

Introduction

Hilot is a traditional healing art of the Philippine Islands. It has been practiced for millennia throughout the 7,000 island archipelago, and is used to heal pain resulting from physical injury. Although the details may vary from region to region, there are underlying principles common throughout the Philippines.

These principles include elements also found in Chinese medicine, such as the balance of opposing forces, and have parallels with some western rehabilitation therapies, including Active Release Therapy (A.R.T.), mayo-fascial release, and Rolfing. Hilot also shares core principles with osteopathic medicine, which is based on achieving a unity of the organism's structure (anatomy) and its functions (physiology). In fact, Hilot shares the four major beliefs that form the foundation of osteopathic medicine:

- the body is a functional unit, an integration of mind, body, and spirit,
- the body can regulate itself, and thus can defend, repair, and remodel itself,
- structure and function are reciprocally interrelated, and
- rational treatment is based on an understanding of body unity, self-regulation, and the interrelationship of structure and function .

The Cohen Method of Soft Tissue Therapy also embraces these four principles. The following is designed to present these techniques and insights in a concise way that will augment hands-on training.

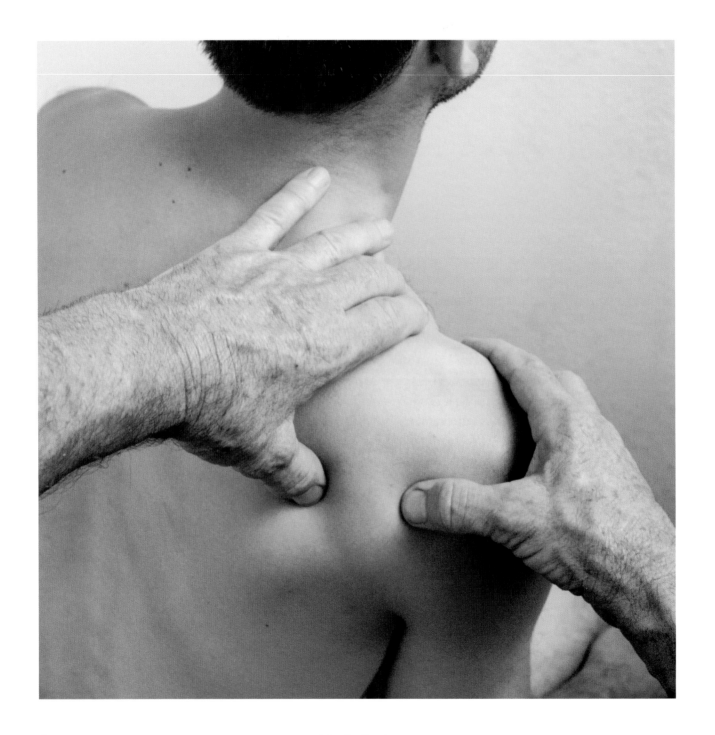

Intentive Touch

At the Root of it All

Fascia

Pain and disease are the body's signals that there is something wrong. Oftentimes, we try to fix the symptoms without looking for the underlying cause. True holistic healing is achieved by looking for the source of the pain and disease while alleviating the symptoms.

"First, let's consider the construction of the human body. One of the most important structural elements is the fascia, which is the biological fabric that holds the body together. You are built of some 70 trillion cells all humming along in relative harmony. The fascia is a three dimensional network of fibrous, wet proteins that hold all the cells in place. The fascial system is a highly complex biomechanical regulatory system, and its proper functioning is crucial to maintaining a dynamic equilibrium between stability and movement. This is essential not only for high performance and recovery from injury, but also for our simple daily life."[2]

"The term "fascia" is increasingly used in scientific and research circles to indicate all of the body's collagen-based soft tissues. This includes all of the tissues labeled "fascia" in classical anatomy as well as all other similar tissues, such as tendons, ligaments, bursae, and the tissues in and around the muscles—endomysium, perimysium, and epimysium. The term also includes the tissues around the organs, such as the coelomic bags that hold the organs in the peritoneum and mesentery in your abdominal cavity and the perineuria membranes that surround the brain, spinal cord, and the peripheral nerves. Some researchers argue that cartilage and bone should be considered fascia."[3]

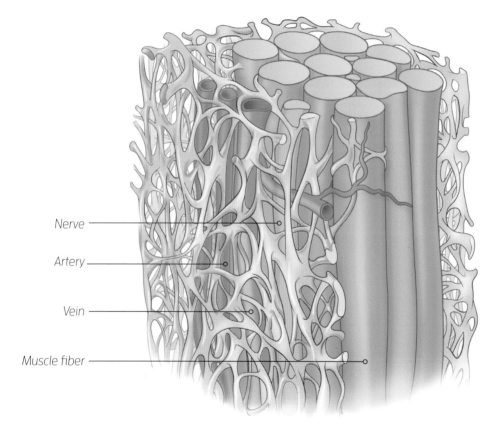

Nerve

Artery

Vein

Muscle fiber

Fig 3.1.1 The fascia network: veins, arteries, nerves

Intentive Touch

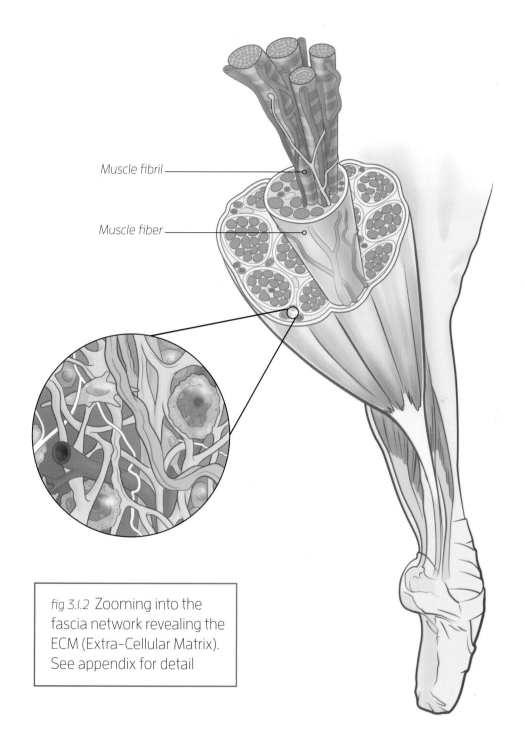

Muscle fibril

Muscle fiber

fig 3.1.2 Zooming into the
fascia network revealing the
ECM (Extra-Cellular Matrix).
See appendix for detail

Overuse

In most cases, pain, discomfort, and injury are rooted in some form of overuse. Many of the overuse-based injuries that I see are the results of social trends that prioritize fitness and body image over a truly healthy, vital body, mind, and spirit. People sometimes use workout regimes designed for highly accomplished athletes in order to push their bodies harder and faster than is appropriate for them. And often, enthusiasm to be active leads many to "go for it" and end up pushing their bodies too hard and too fast. This is known as the Weekend Warrior Syndrome—the attempt to get in shape through irregular, intensive bursts of untrained exercise rather than through consistent workouts. In other words, it is what happens when you don't exercise at all during the week and then overdo your exercise on the weekend.

Another leading cause of overuse-related injuries is a lack of exercise. This sneaks up on people as they age. While most people's youths are carefree and active, adulthood introduces many more tasks. The pressure of the school years transitions into the working world of adulthood, including responsibilities that range from pursuing a career to caring for elderly relatives and starting families. The change occurs gradually and even imperceptibly, but the prevalence of desk jobs, chronic cell phone use, and a lack of bodily self-awareness have created a vast array of new aches and pains in our population. This overuse not only affects our physical bodies, but the mental, emotional, and spiritual aspects of our lives as well.

Overusing the muscles, whether through improper exercise, work, or other stresses, causes them to tighten until they become extremely stiff. As a result, they don't move as freely as when relaxed, causing the muscle tissue to become matted together. When this happens, the life force is unable to flow properly through the connective tissues of the biological fabric, causing imbalance, dysfunction, and pain. You can picture this phenomenon as a traffic jam in your body. This congestion causes the musculo-skeletal system to work out of sync just enough to cause small contractions near the place where the the muscle-tendon attaches to the bone. Because the body is extremely adaptable, it will compensate for this blockage by finding new ways to move. These adaptive patterns of movement are often less efficient and can ultimately develop spasms, pulled muscles, strains, sprains, and accompanying inflammation.

Dehydration

One major hidden source of injury is dehydration. Our bodies are approximately 60-70% water[4]. When that volume is decreased, there is a corresponding decrease in the amount of oxygen in the blood. This affects the flow of electrical impulses along our nerves and makes our soft tissues denser, inhibiting the flow of the life force through connective tissues, which inhibits the body's self-regulating mechanisms. This can lead to cramping and or pulled and torn muscles.

The good news is that one of the best ways to prevent injury is simply to stay hydrated. The best way to do that is to sip water or other hydrating liquids throughout the day, rather than gulping down large volumes at long intervals. Gulping doesn't allow the cells to absorb the water, and often the water just passes through the body.

Poor Posture and Uneven Breathing

When we concentrate on work or study for long periods of time, we often unknowingly adopt a poor posture and uneven breathing patterns that cause repetitive stress symptoms that, in turn, lead to pain as well as to inefficient work.

Unrecognized uneven breathing patterns often develop into the habit of holding your breath. This happens often if you are doing something new or difficult, such as an athletic movement, lifting something awkward or heavy, or doing intricate or close work. When you hold your breath, the pressure of the fluid surrounding your spinal cord and brain, intrathecal pressure, is increased[5]. Over time, an increase in this pressure can increase your risk of herniating a disc in your spine. Holding your breath also creates tension in your rib cage, engaging the diaphragm. On the other hand, continuous and even breathing reduces intrathecal pressure, leaving enough room for free movement without the irritation that can lead to a protective reactive response.

There are simple measures you can take to address this: Breathe evenly and sip water (or other hydrating beverages) at frequent and regular intervals to stay refreshed. Get up frequently to give your body a break from static positioning and to allow your blood to flow through your body. Check your ergonomics often to make sure you aren't stuck in an awkward position. These check-ins create short breaks from work and add significant quality to daily routines, especially in times of high stress.

The Protective Reactive Response

Often an initial injury, caused by a slip or a fall or a twist of an ankle, becomes chronic because the body compensates. How does this happen? An initial tweak from a sudden or awkward movement, or from overuse and fatigue, causes a spasm in the surrounding soft tissues. This affects the kinetic chain—the series of successive tissues and joints that constitute a complex motor unit—and activates the body's protective reactive response. The protective reactive response is a byproduct of the stretch reflex, which is activated when an increased load on a joint puts pressure on the surrounding connective and muscle tissues. The body's response is to put the area on "high alert." In order to prevent injury, a proprioceptive mechanism—the body's way of protecting itself—goes into action, contracting to stabilize the musculo-tendon near its attachment to the bone and relaxing the opposing muscle to maintain balance. The tendon is designed to return to its original length and tension once the load is normalized. However, it sometimes doesn't, and the result is imbalance, spasms, pain, and dysfunction.

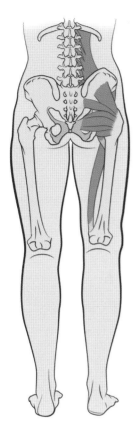

fig 3.5.1 Muscles released into a neutral position

Example of kinetic chain reaction along the hip when irregulariy occurs

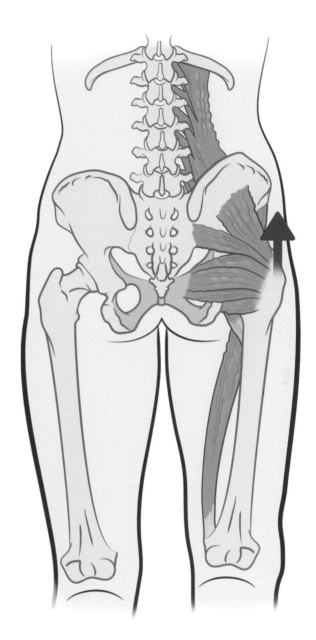

fig 3.5.2 Muscles in contracted state

The reason it doesn't return to its original length involves the proper delivery of nutrient-rich blood to nerve proprioceptors called golgi tendon organs (which reports changes in muscle tension) and the spindle cell, which reports changes in muscle length. When the spindle cell is stretched, it tells the muscle to contract and the opposing muscle to relax.[6] If the soft tissues become traumatized, the smooth muscle lining of the blood vessels constricts, especially near this proprioceptive mechanism. This reduces the blood flow, which in turn reduces the ability of the nerve impulses to "reboot" the stretch reflex. In other words, the stretch reflex can't return the tendon to its original neutral resting state, which would relax the constriction of the soft tissues around the joint.

In short, pain can have its roots in anything from traumatic injury to the way you sit at the computer—and all can trigger the protective reactive response. Add dehydration and uneven breathing into the mix, and suddenly that seemingly mysterious pain doesn't seem so mysterious anymore.

But there is hope.

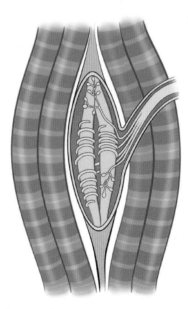

fig 3.5.3 Relaxed / neutral spindle cell

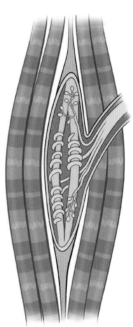

fig 3.5.4 Stretched spindle cell

Intentive Touch

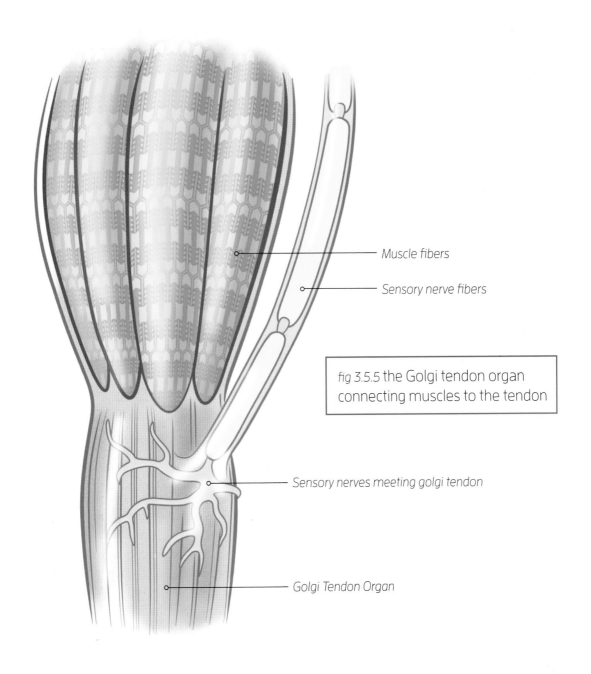

Muscle fibers

Sensory nerve fibers

fig 3.5.5 the Golgi tendon organ connecting muscles to the tendon

Sensory nerves meeting golgi tendon

Golgi Tendon Organ

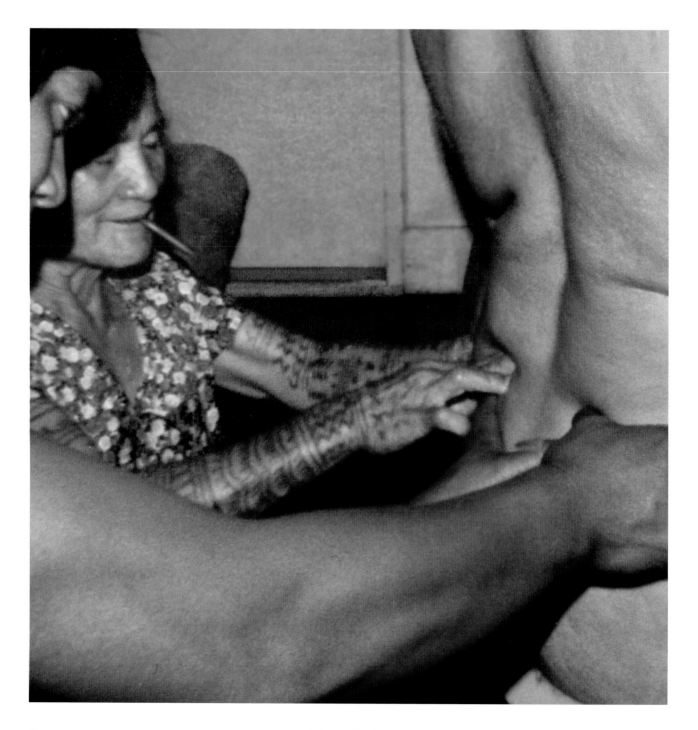

Intentive Touch

Introduction to Hilot

Hilot,[7] the Filipino art of therapeutic massage, has been helping people with such conditions for literally thousands of years. Traditionally passed down orally, it is one of many categories of folk medicine. The full gamut of Filipino folk doctors includes herbalists, bone setters, obstetricians, and other specialists such as snake– or animal– bite curers, as well as shamans or spiritual healers. All of their practices share roots with other South Asian and Southeast Asian healing traditions.

A Hilot practitioner is called a manghihilot. The ability to heal is seen, above all, as a gift, and manghihilots pass this gift on to others out of gratitude rather than for gain. They believe in a greater source of power or healing energy and see themselves as healing instruments. They believe that the physical and spiritual worlds are entwined, though their philosophy of healing may be based in either science or spirituality, or both.

Theory and Benefits

Many people in the Philippines believe that in addition to the strictly physical causes of pain outlined above, illness and physical disability may be caused by encounters with bad or disturbed spirits. In such cases, the affected person might make an offering or pray to a higher power. For healers who use massage, the massage may be used to drive away a spirit that has lodged itself in the affected person.

In Hilot, on both metaphysical and physical levels, the concept of pasma (imbalance) from exposure to extreme temperatures, from hot to cold or cold to hot, plays an important role. Any sudden contrast of temperature within the body or the spirit compromises vigor, making the body susceptible to illness.

"The channels that carry spiritual energy, called 'urat' and 'pennet,' also play a very important role, and unblocking these channels is the primary goal of Hilot. The terms urat and pennet also refer to nerves, veins, tendons, arteries, sinews, ligaments, muscles, intestines, the windpipe, and other such structures. All of these can be visualized as channel- or tube-like structures through which anything can pass, including blood, air, food, water, plasma, sweat, lymph, nerve impulses, and the life force. A number of other cultures share the concept of such channels, including those of India, Thailand, Indonesia, Malaysia, Micronesia, and Polynesia.

A blockage in one or more of these channels is like the congestion described above. This blockage can be caused by the displacement or compression of the blood vessels and nerves, as well as by an imbalance of hot and cold or by a spiritual disruption."[8]

According to Ina Facucad, the blood vessels have a smooth muscle lining that constricts when there is a disturbance, injury, or imbalance.[9] This restricts the flow of blood, nerve impulses, and the life force, which in turn restricts the distribution of nutrients and the elimination of waste. If nutrients aren't delivered and waste is not eliminated, the nerves can't function properly. The constriction of the vessel lining also prevents connective tissues from stretching and gliding smoothly against each other. This can eventually cause various structures, especially the channels (urat and pennet), to compress, atrophy, and adhere to one another, creating a cycle in which congestion leads to more congestion.

Improving the circulation of the blood is a key goal in Hilot, and parallels the tradition in Chinese medicine "in which blood is the mother of chi, and chi is the commander of blood," with chi understood as the life-force (see appendix for detail). Blood and chi are inherently connected, and the proper flow of blood and the life-force is what enables self-healing. Working together, they allow the body to regain its proper balance. By decongesting the channels through which blood and energy flow, the mayo-fascial (muscle and connective) tissues, as well as all the other organs fed by the channels, are in turn decongested. Massage softens tissues and encourages improved circulation, thus enabling the blood and life-force to supply the nutrients needed to heal the body.

Hilot benefits both the giver and the receiver. The manghihilot, attentive in both mind and spirit, accesses a oneness with the world through practicing this gift, while the client is relieved from tension and pain and enjoys improved circulation through the blood, lymph, eliminatory, respiratory, and nervous systems.

According to Philippine tradition, the client must willingly accept the gift of Hilot; if he or she has any doubts about the method, the therapy will not be effective, no matter how excellent the work. Strong results depend upon trust, a feeling of oneness, and a sense of caring and love.

Application

To summarize: the fundamental goal of Hilot is to free up compressed, compacted, and/or tangled vascular tissue within the neurovascular bundle (the sheath housing the blood vessels and nerves), though this does not necessarily mean that the manghihilot literally tracks individual vessels. Instead, and unique to Hilot, the practitioner's touch travels along the connective tissues' fascial fabric, as if that fabric were fiber-optic filaments, transferring information, energy, and nutrients to compromised soft tissues, releasing them from their protective reactivity. The process dilates the blood vessels, returning them to their normal size. When this occurs, the dynamic relationship between blood and the life-force is effectively rebooted and returned to its normal balance [10].

The manghihilot begins by patiently observing the subject and noting how the elements (heat, cold, wind, and damp) affect the subject's condition. S/he will then begin to warm up the tissue in order to avoid shocking the body with deep pressure. This warming, along with an examination of the range of motion, gives the practitioner the information s/he needs to best address the area of concern. S/he will then stroke across the muscle fibers, moving away from the heart, to begin to open up the channels. The manghihilot will also check for blockages or stiffness in areas that directly or indirectly correspond to the injured body part, working along that path to open it up. The manghihilot uses coconut or sesame oil to increase the fingers' sensitivity when manipulating the urat, or the muscle and connective tissues, or both.

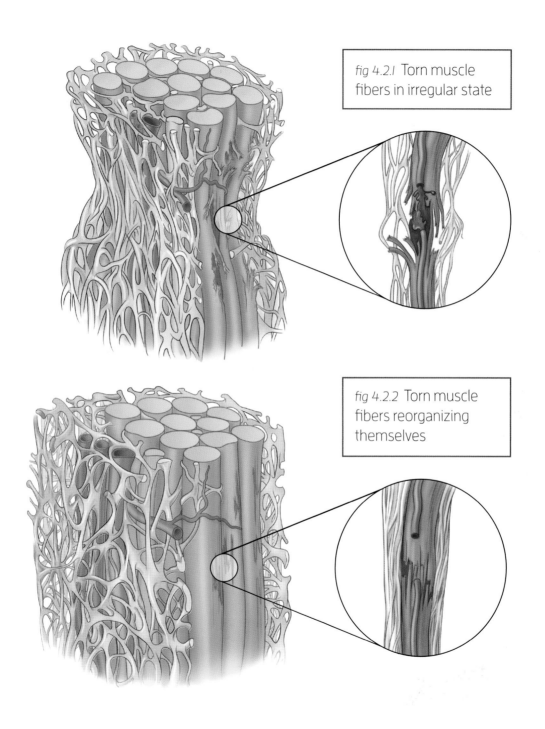

fig 4.2.1 Torn muscle fibers in irregular state

fig 4.2.2 Torn muscle fibers reorganizing themselves

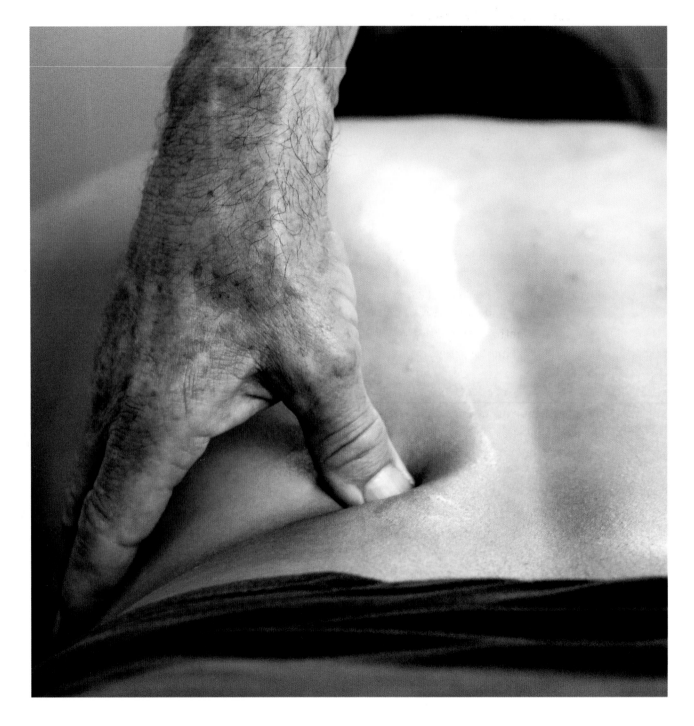

Intentive Touch

Introduction to Intentive Touch

Investigative Touch and Engaged Touch

There are several ways that these healing traditions are passed on. Sometimes they are transferred from parent to child; sometimes they are revealed in dreams, and sometimes they are passed on to someone outside the community. This was the way that I learned.

When I first arrived in the Philippines, I was fascinated by the new and unusual environment. It had all my senses heightened, and this was accentuated by the need to care for my brother in this foreign land, a process that took me, through touch and feel, into the universal and timeless realms of the healing process.

This fascination created the discipline I needed to take the training from the Philippine masters, along with thirty-five years of subsequent study and hands-on experience, and develop it into my own practice and method, which I have termed Intentive Touch. Every therapeutic method is distinguished by its unique touch.

The distinguishing feature of Intentive Touch is the quality of the touch itself. It combines attention, invention, intention, intensity, and intervention. Intentive Touch occurs in two stages: Investigative Touch and Engaged Touch.

Investigative Touch includes the stages of examination and analysis—this is when, in consultation with your client, you come to an understanding of the problem and determine the best course of therapy.

Engaged Touch is the healing component. As you begin Engaged Touch, maintain the investigative component to help you stay focused. Use it to balance the resistance of the soft tissues in the subject's affected area(s) around the contact point. This contact point is usually your thumbs or fingers, but in cases in which more leverage or pressure is needed, an elbow, knee, or foot might be used. Balancing, in this sense, means applying pressure to encourage or persuade the stretch reflex to "reset," thereby rebalancing the density of the soft tissue.

During the session, both Investigative and Engaged Touch are constantly and simultaneously in play.

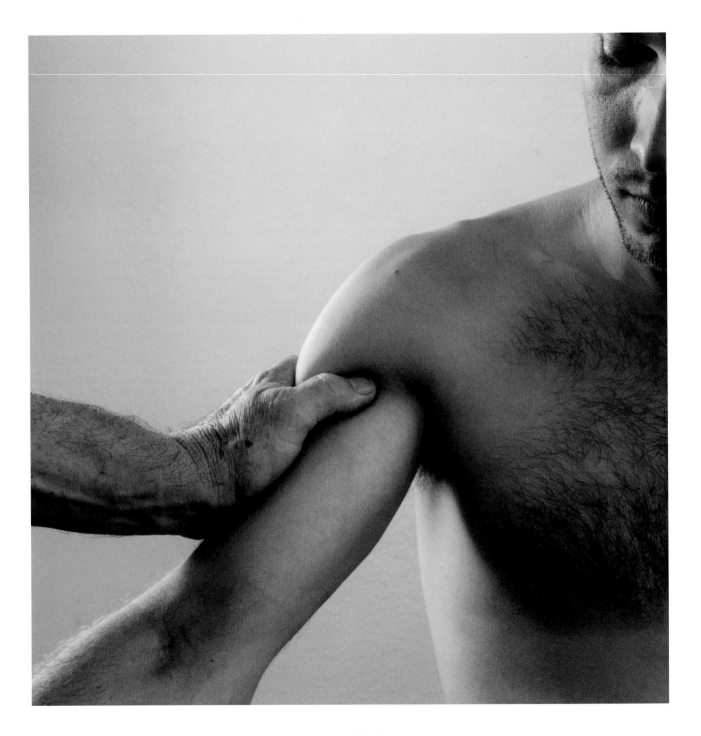

Intentive Touch

Getting Started

Observe

When you observe, you open up and take in, without resistance or preconceptions, and observation begins the moment you meet your subject. How is s/he breathing? How is s/he standing? What do you notice in the posture? As you become attuned, you'll start being able to see symptoms of imbalance in the soft tissues even before you touch the subject.

Observe not only how your subjects move, but also how they speak and how their facial expressions change. Listen to the content of the supposed "chit chat" during the session—what is it really about? And all the while, observe how it's affecting you. This initial observation is crucial and should become the ritual with which you begin every session, no matter how well you know the subject.

You will notice that your state of mind changes when you're with a subject. Observe how you feel when you hold the subject; pay close attention to your impressions, intuitions, and observations. The more you observe, the more you have to work with.

Observe the subject standing in a relaxed position, then walking, and then seated; these various modes will allow you to collect impressions from different perspectives and begin to gather them into an overall assessment, while you also get a sense of how the subject is responding to you.

Always remember that, in this line of work, your subjects are not feeling their best. People in pain can be impatient, irritable, and just plain difficult, which can make for poor communication, compromising the outcome. Keeping this in mind and always treating your subjects with compassion are among your most important tools. In turn, they'll find comfort in your bedside manner, which will relax them and lead to a more effective treatment.

After this initial exchange of impressions, you'll need to prepare your subject for the actual therapy.

Create a Comfortable Setting

The physical environment in which you conduct your therapy sessions is important; it is through it, as well as through your demeanor, that the subject gets his or her first impression of you. Everything in the environment needs to establish and reinforce the sense of confidence necessary for your subjects to trust their bodies in your hands. Make sure that all sheets and pillow cases are always fresh and clean, and that the environment as a whole is both clean and clutter-free. Clarity in the session room helps both practitioner and subject stay calm and focused. Think carefully about what, if anything, you hang on the walls—what conscious and sub-conscious messages might your images give? Extend this critical attention to all the objects in the room—the books, the plants, the mementos—make sure they all work together to create a healthful and harmonious whole. Make sure that the air is fresh, but draft-free, as exposure to drafts, especially cold ones, can have a negative effect on the body. Also make sure that both light and temperature are adjustable—some people thrive on light, while others are calmed by a dimmer atmosphere. I suggest using defused natural spectrum light that can be easily adjusted by a rheostat. Similarly, people have different temperature preferences. Since temperature cannot be adjusted as quickly as light can, you might want to ask your subjects about their temperature preferences when the appointment is made. Music or other background sound is also a crucial element of ambiance; many practitioners choose not to use background music, as it can interfere with concentration and a peaceful calm. If you do use music, always give subjects the option of having it turned off or of choosing the style and volume. Other options for background sound include ambient natural sounds, such as that of waves or light wind. Being able to adjust these parameters to your subjects' comfort lets them know that you are thinking holistically and that they are your first priority.

Modesty

How much clothing (if any) your subjects wear must be left up to them. Even if a given procedure would be easier and more efficient with the clothing removed, because levels of modesty differ widely, honoring your subjects' preferences in this area is key to their relaxed and receptive attitude.

Positioning the Body – Part A

The last stage of preparation requires positioning your subject's body for Investigative Touch. This is the explorative stage, in which you determine the nature of the condition; you will reposition your subject's body for the healing step of Engaged Touch, and we'll cover that in detail below.

For Investigative Touch, position the body so that it is loose and comfortable, allowing you free access to the area(s) in question. Though each situation will dictate a specific positioning, there are some general principles to keep in mind. Think of the body as a kinetic chain—the head is connected to the neck and shoulders, the neck and shoulders are connected to the arms and back, the back is connected to the hip and legs etc.—and pressure put on one part will affect the next and so on. Be aware of this chain, and make sure that the body parts both "downstream" and "upstream" of the place you're working on are comfortably and freely positioned. For example, if you're working on the shoulder, make sure that the arm is comfortably in a neutral position and not being inadvertently strained. Or if you are working on the upper back, make sure that the neck isn't compromised, causing tension and possible stiffness without your knowing. Remaining constantly aware of how your subject is responding to your touch is the best way to avoid such inadvertent strains.

You are now ready to begin Investigative Touch.

Applying Touch

The first step of Investigative Touch is to extend your observations from your eyes to your fingers, paying close attention to what you feel when you hold the body. Be aware of the density of the soft tissues under your fingers—how dense are they compared to the tissues around them? Are they contracted or in spasm (hard)? Or dehydrated? Don't be concerned if you can't distinguish these things at first. Consistent attention will increasingly sensitize you to these differences.

Continue your tactile observation, comparing various body parts and tissues—do some tissues feel spongy or stringy? Are there inconsistencies in some places, places that feel different from the tissues surrounding them? Sometimes the skin itself will also give clues. Its feel can range from slippery, tacky, slimy, and sweaty to dry, abrasive, and flaky. As your fingers become more sensitized to these differences, you'll begin to receive the messages they're sending you.

What you're looking and feeling for with Investigative Touch is an area in the fabric of the soft tissues that is uncommonly dense. The muscle may feel taut or tight, or it may feel full. Imagine a balloon filled with water; if the balloon is only partially full, the fluid will move away when you push on it, but if it's completely full, there's nowhere for the water to go, and your pressure will meet with resistance. This resistance is caused by the muscle fibers' contracting during the stretch reflex and then not releasing. Such contraction without release is often the underlying cause of the injury. Because they are overloaded, the muscles haven't been allowed to self-regulate, which is to say, release and re-lengthen after contraction. This potential for resistance is particularly important to keep in mind during Engaged Touch.

The bodily area offering the most resistance is often not the area where your subject is feeling the most pain, and yet often that's where your work needs to begin because that's where the blockage can begin to dissolve. Once you have noted these areas through Investigative Touch, it's time for Engaged Touch to begin.

But first, the body must be repositioned based upon the information you've gleaned from your Investigative Touch.

Positioning the Body — Part B

Again, think of the body as a kinetic chain; this chain is disrupted by the body's compensatory response to injury—in other words, when injured, the body will change the way it moves in order to save the injured area from pressure, work, or strain.

Although there is no set way to position the body, there are general principles to guide you. The basic options for positioning your subject on a therapy table include sitting or lying down; if lying down, you must then choose from lying face up, face down, or on one side.

Decide between sitting and lying down based, first, on which position gives you the easiest and widest range of access to the areas of resistant density that you located during Investigative Touch and, second, on which is most comfortable for your subject. And, in fact, that second often comes first, as being flexible with positioning is key to establishing trust; it tells subjects that you put their feelings first and will, above all, not do anything to hurt them. I find that people are willing to follow my suggestions for positioning once trust is established.

One general principle: Remember gravity! Gravity causes some of the vascular and connective tissues to settle deep into the layers of muscle and the biological fabric of the extra cellular matrix, making it hard to get to them, particularly when the subject is lying face down.

If the problem is in the neck, shoulders, back, or chest, a sitting position will quite likely be best, though having your subject lie face up can offer access to certain areas of the neck and upper shoulder. Having your subject lie face up often also works well for issues in the legs and hips, or when lying face down causes lower back pain. When working on the back itself, you can position your subject sitting or lying face up, face down, or on one side, depending on the part of the back you're treating.

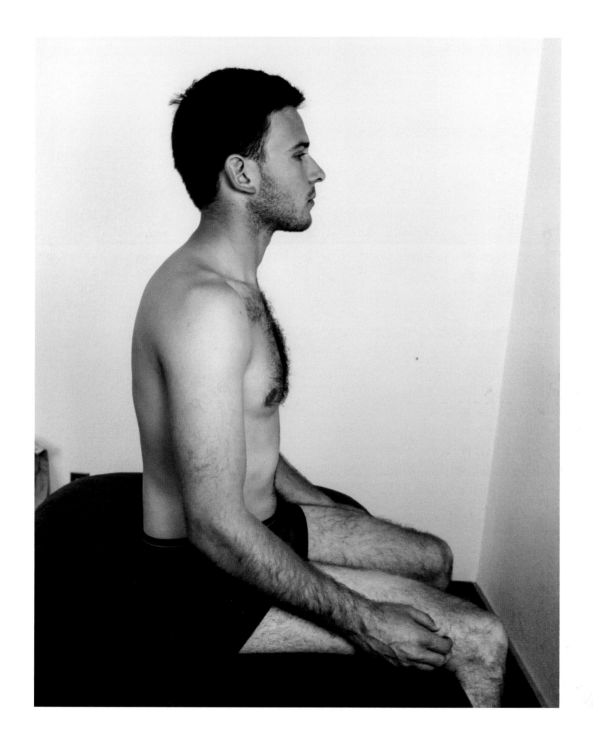

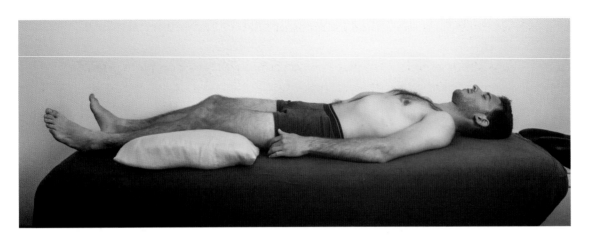

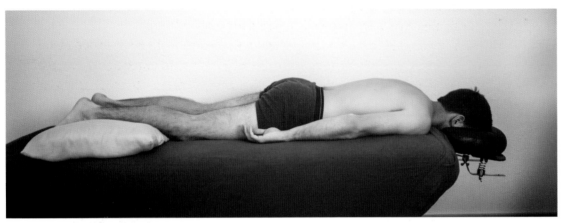

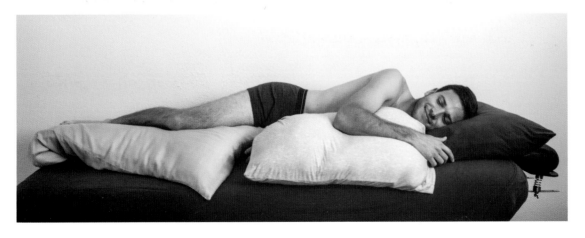

Intentive Touch

Other things to keep in mind for repositioning the body during sessions:

-   A sitting position can give you access to a soft tissue problem that you
    might miss if the subject is lying down. When seated, be sure that your
    subject's feet are solidly touching the ground, so that the whole body is
    stable and your touch doesn't throw it off-balance.
-   Lying face down works best when a sitting position would aggravate
    painful stiffness, tightness, and/or spasm in the muscles. A lying-down
    position allows you to feel where muscle tissue that should be at rest is
    actually still engaged, making it possible to directly address what may be
    the source of the problem. However, if the problem is caused by over-
    extension in the spine from contracted protective reactivity, then having
    your subject lie face down can aggravate this condition.
-   Having your subject lie face up is the best position when lower back pain
    is strong, as it relieves the spinal extension caused by the reactive tightness
    to the surrounding muscle groups, the hamstrings, and those in the front
    of the hip.
-   Having your subject lie on one side is particularly good for working on the
    hip area, which includes the spine, pelvis, femur, and all the soft tissues that
    connect these parts with others in the kinetic chain. This position also allows
    access to the quadratus lumborum, the muscle that connects the pelvis to
    the spine and the lowest ribs. This is often a key to unblocking disturbances
    in the kinetic chain between the upper and lower parts of the body.

You are now ready to begin Engaged Touch.

Keeping in mind an image of the dynamic nature of the biological fascial fabric will help your fingers to "see" as you intuitively stroke along the direction of the fibers of the tissues [11]. In natural movements, muscle contractions are multifaceted; the fibers get confused when they are overloaded, resulting in the area's becoming static, like a computer that has frozen up and needs to be rebooted [12]. As the overloaded muscle fibers contract, density develops until it feels like a cord adhering to the biological fabric around it. It has a ropey quality like that of a washcloth or small towel that has been wrung out and then dried. When you encounter a dense area, slightly release, and then apply a bit more pressure, then stop, but remain in contact. From the point of contact, you will feel a slight channel that your finger or thumb will define as you continue to move away from the initial contact point. Continue to follow this, and you will be creating the path of myofascial release for that area of density.

Gradually, you'll learn to identify and isolate the precise point at which the pressure you're applying meets the point of greatest resistance and density—this is where the healing begins. Maintain contact with this area while slightly releasing the pressure, allowing the tissue around the point of contact to respond to the resistant pressure it has encountered. There will be a subtle change in resistance; it will feel as if a cord-like grouping of resistant fibers is melting and reintegrating into the soft tissues surrounding it. This reintegration allows the proper flow of the life force to resume.

In summary: The stroking/releasing gesture is the core of Engaged Touch, and its purpose is to open up blocked channels. Keep in mind that this is an act of communication; you are, in effect, "telling" the muscle fibers and associated tissues to respond, but in order to do this, the connective tissues' fascial fabric carrying the command signals along their networks must be open and unobstructed. If there is too much density within the muscle fibers, the message simply cannot get through correctly, which causes dysfunctions such as tightness, muscle spasms, and inflammation.

There is a mental parallel to this physical engagement, and that is your belief and your intention to resolve and repair, in short, to heal, the disturbance that you identified during Investigative Touch.

Staying in Touch

I find it helpful to maintain a level of light verbal contact throughout the session, asking from time to time "How are you?" or "Are you ok?" This offers a non-committal invitation for the subject's response and input and assures that you are present and connected to him or her. Some people are quiet during a session, even if they are experiencing pain. However, the old adage of "no pain, no gain" is not always correct; keep in touch with the subject's immediate sensations, so that you can gauge the level of his or her pain and adjust your touch accordingly.

It's also important to keep in communication so that subjects do not "check out," wandering from their bodies, making them unable to supply the input that could direct the therapy to a positive outcome. Keep your subjects' personalities in mind and modulate the tone and pitch of your voice as well as the frequency and energy of your comments to meet them where they are most comfortable.

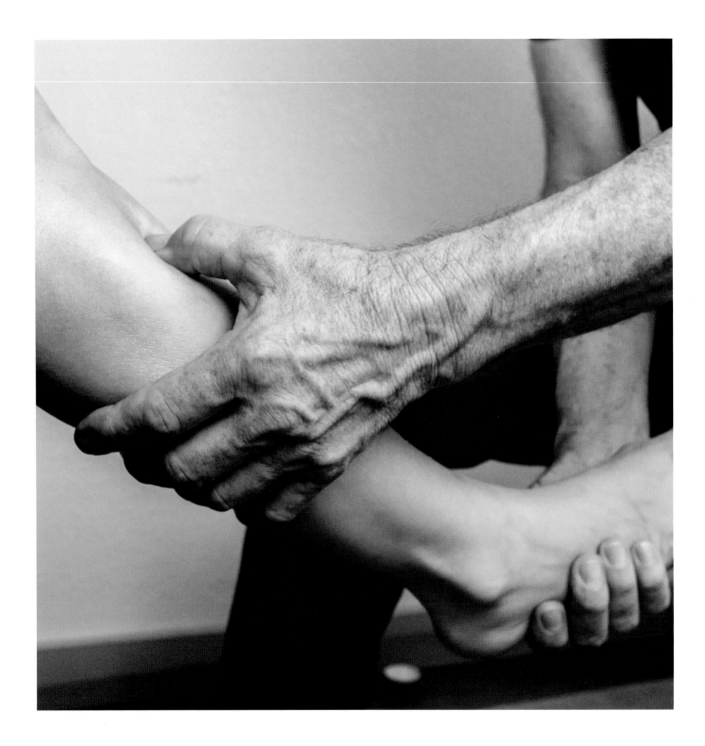

Developing Intentive Touch

As I mentioned above, with consistent, attentive practice, your fingers will learn to "listen" and "see"—and it really is as if they add these concrete senses to their tactile capacities. But there are also techniques that can help you develop a sense of different tissue qualities and recognize the "geography" of body tissue in general.

Intentive Touch can be compared to a search and rescue mission. The Investigative component is the search and the Engaged component, when the fixing takes place, is the rescue.

I find it important to remember that when the density of the soft tissues increases, the probability of dysfunction increases. As you come to recognize this, your touch will increasingly be able to release the density within the given area, and your feel for this release will develop more and more over time.

Peeling an Orange

Consider the orange: its components are remarkably similar to the tissues in our bodies. The peel is like the layers of our skin, and the white, which surrounds the entire peeled fruit as well as each individual section, is like our bodies' fascial fabric. The sections themselves are similar to our muscle groups in their fascial coverings. The juicy part is actually individual cells filled with juice, and they are analogous to our muscle fibers. The juice only spills out of the fruit if you tear the membrane. Don't. Practice taking the entire fruit apart without letting a single drop of juice escape. Peeling the fruit and separating the sections slowly and carefully feels similar to treating a dense area in the body with Engaged Touch. Practice until you can get the entire skin off of an orange intact.

Coming Unglued

The second practice technique is similar in that it develops your feel for peeling matted tissues apart. Take contact cement and spread it onto the surface of various objects, such as a citrus fruit, a plastic bottle, and a piece of wood or bamboo. Spread a patch about four inches square over the surface, leave it long enough to get tacky, and then with your thumb proceed to loosen it and gently peel it off the surface. Practice until you can get it up in a single piece with no tears.

Both of these techniques allow you to practice separating matted soft tissues.

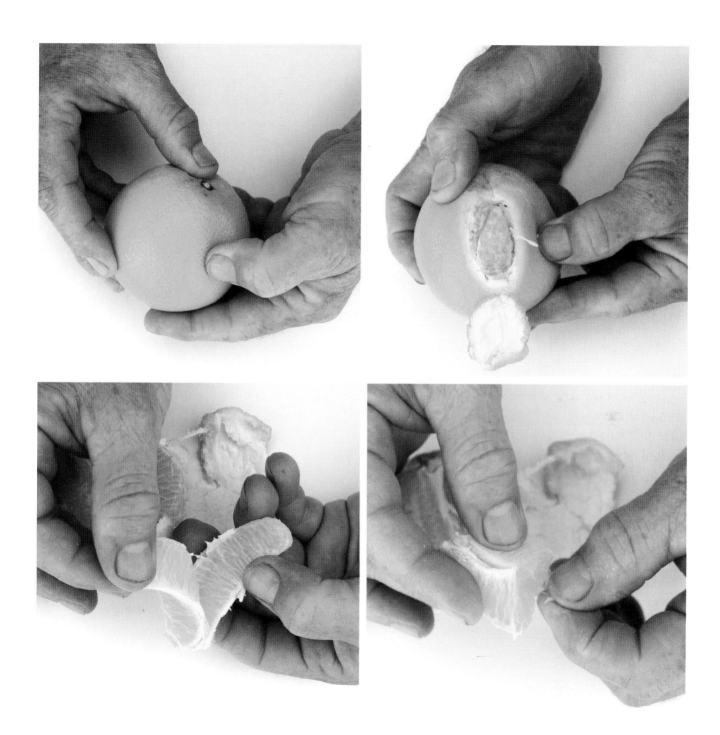

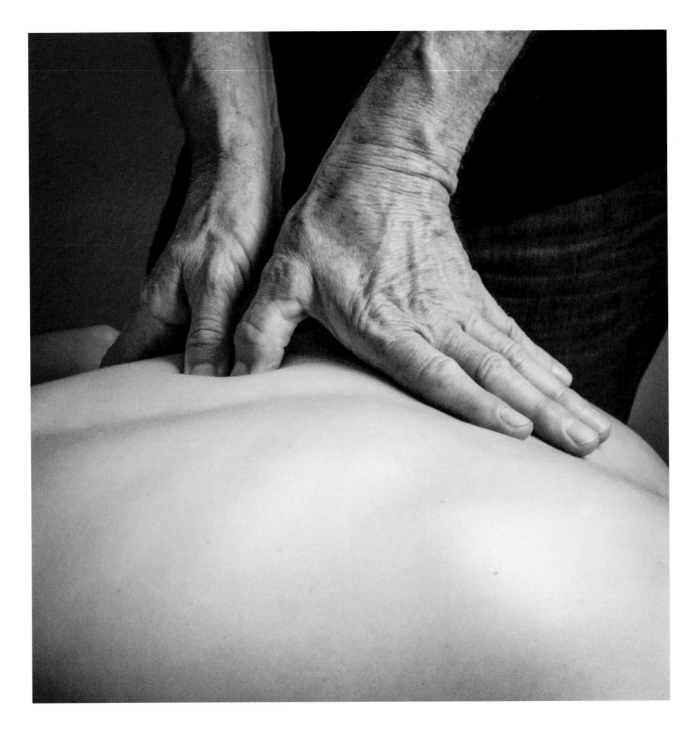

Intentive Touch

Frequently Injured Areas

Every injury is as unique as the person injured, which means that a book such as this can't possibly address all the injuries you'll encounter in your subjects, but taking a moment to trace the cause and treatment of a few specific examples may give you a map for approaching your own subjects.

Some areas, by their very natures, are more frequently injured than others; these include the complex joints that get a lot of use, such as shoulders and hips, and the "energy intersections," such as the lower back—places where energies from various parts of the body cross on their way to other zones. While, again, each injury is unique, there are general issues to keep in mind that will help you address each of these challenging areas.

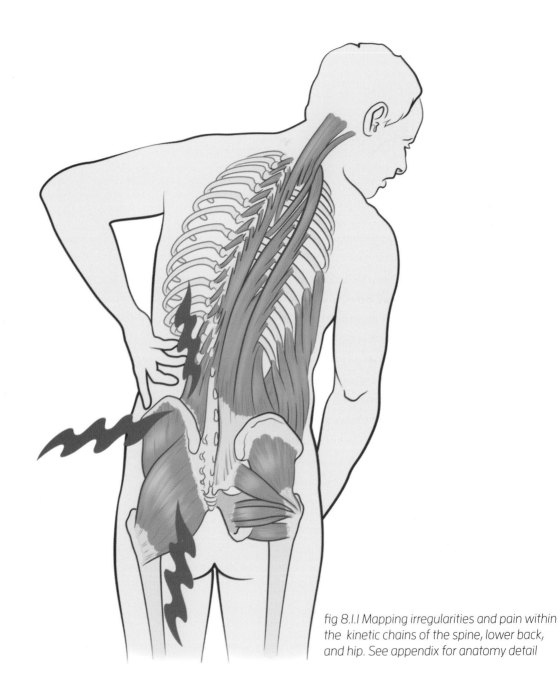

fig 8.1.1 Mapping irregularities and pain within the kinetic chains of the spine, lower back, and hip. See appendix for anatomy detail

Intentive Touch

Hip

I recently treated an otherwise healthy 56-year-old man who had overstretched his hip area (hip flexors, gluteus muscles, and hamstrings). He came to me explaining that he had recently taken up a strenuous exercise routine in order to get in shape for a rugged backpacking trip coming up in the summer. The routine had proved a bit too strenuous, and he found himself unable to bend forward without pain. This caused muscle spasms that, in turn, limited the disk space in his spine. Without enough space to move freely, the spinal nerves became irritated and inflamed. Within a couple of weeks, the situation had aggravated into a bulging disc that caused extreme pain in his lower leg.

An epidural injection of corticosteroids reduced the inflammation at the nerve roots around the protruding disc, and after a few days, he was able to move with less pain in his lower leg, but he still was very stiff, and he could not walk normally.

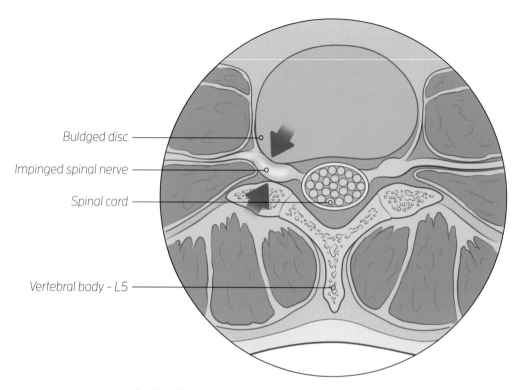

Buldged disc

Impinged spinal nerve

Spinal cord

Vertebral body - L5

fig 8.I.2 Cross section of L-5 with bulging disc and spinal nerve impingement

After a thorough examination with Investigative Touch, I decided that the best approach was to release the contraction in the muscles around his hip (the pelvis, upper leg, and lumbar spine) in order to relieve the residual pressure on the spinal nerves that had been caused by the protective reactive response to the nerve irritation. I used Engaged Touch on these areas, applying pressure until I felt the resistance subside. I continued with similar strokes overlapping above and below, working from the C7 vertebra to the L5, including the lumbo-sacral joint. I then applied pressure with my thumb at the base of the last rib and stroked with exploratory firmness until I felt the border of the quadratus lumborum and continued to the outer ridge of the iliac crest where the quadratus lumborum attaches.

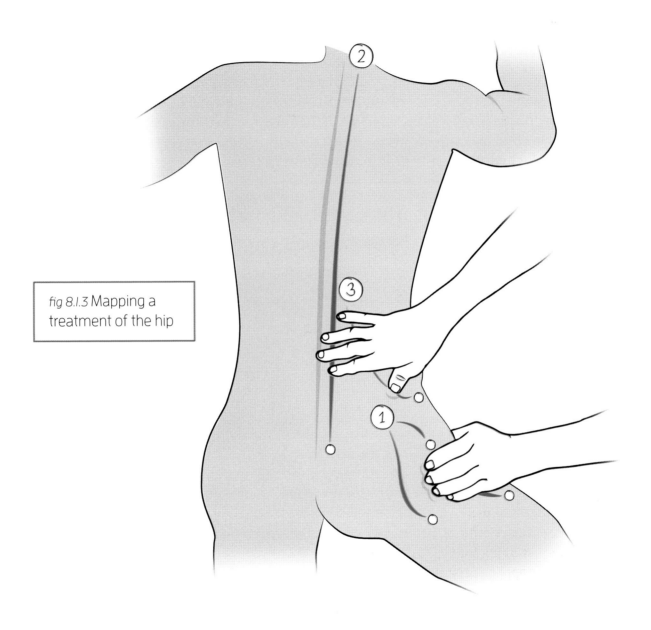

fig 8.1.3 Mapping a treatment of the hip

Releasing the contractions in these muscles created more clearance for the moving parts, resulting in less irritation to the nerves because the peripheral nerve reactivity, which keeps the muscles contracted and limits blood flow to the spindle cell/golgi tendon, had calmed down to normal. This had the effect of "rebooting" the proprioceptive mechanism of the stretch reflex, returning the spindle cell to its most neutral position. In other words, the area was back in balance, not only able to move smoothly and correctly, but also primed to protect itself in the case of further stress. This achieved a quick resolution of the muscular dysfunction and allowed him to use his hip muscles correctly. He left the session commenting on how light his leg felt and walking normally for the first time in weeks.

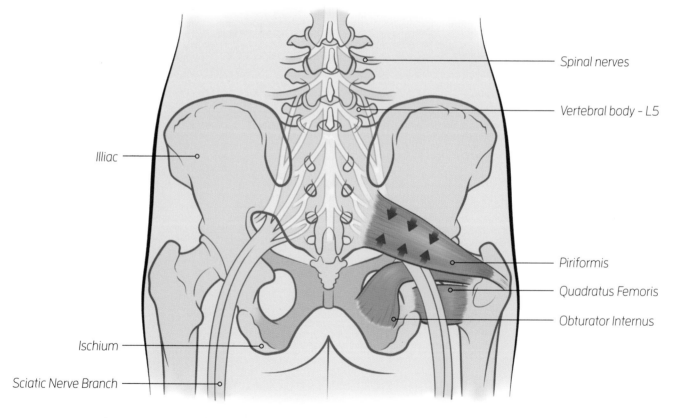

fig 8.1.5 Posterior view of pelvic girdle with external rotator muscles and sciatic nerve branch

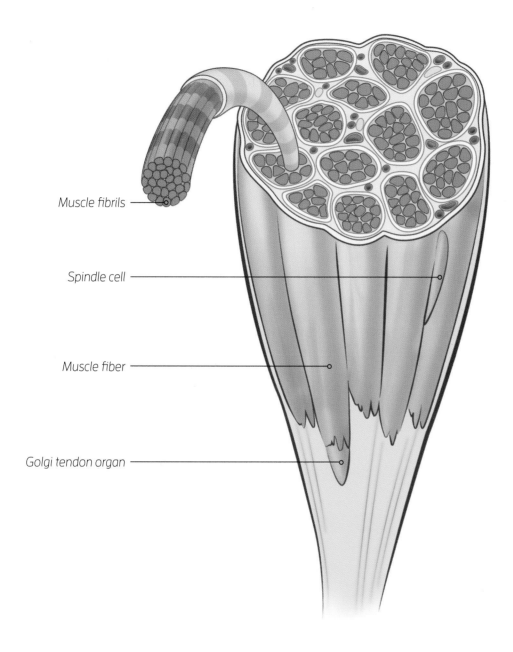

Muscle fibrils

Spindle cell

Muscle fiber

Golgi tendon organ

fig 8.1.6 Cross section of tendon at muscle junction

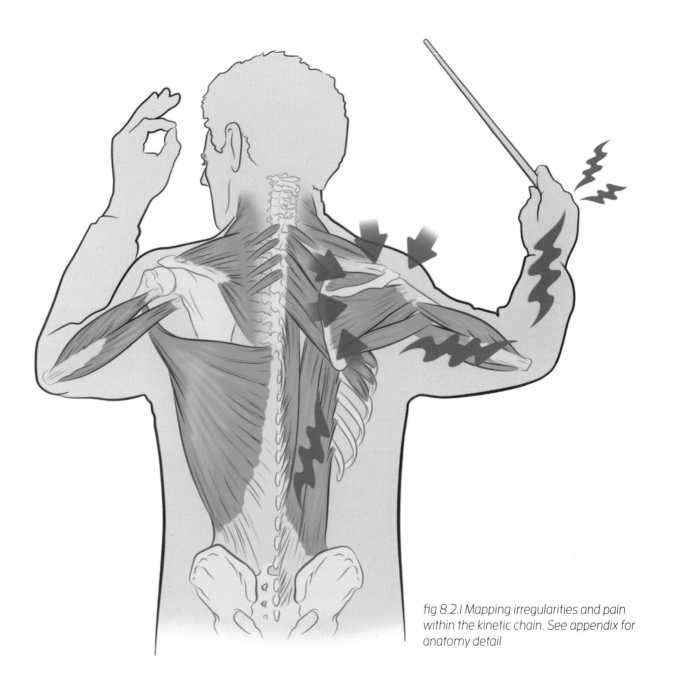

fig 8.2.1 Mapping irregularities and pain within the kinetic chain. See appendix for anatomy detail

Intentive Touch

Shoulder

The shoulder is a very unusual joint in that it is only attached to the skeleton where the clavicle meets the sternum—so it's floating out there without much support. And we use it all the time—and some of us more than others. An internationally prominent orchestra conductor, aging like the rest of us, has been a subject of mine for the past 10 years. He has chronic right shoulder pain that at times extends to his arm and hand and affects his ability to hold the baton properly. The problem fluctuates from mild stiffness to extreme pain, depending on how much traveling and performing he's doing.

He came to me recently after an international tour of several weeks, during which, unfortunately, he'd slipped and fallen backward, breaking his fall by grabbing a doorknob with his right arm, which no doubt prevented what could have been a serious injury, but aggravated his chronic condition. When he arrived in my office, he was experiencing referred pain throbbing from the top back of his shoulder down to his ring and pinky fingers. It was particularly acute when he was lying down, and so woke him up throughout the night.

An MRI revealed some minor tears in and around the shoulder girdle, but it was unclear whether they were recent or from previous wear and tear. With only a few days before he was due to travel to Europe to guest-conduct—and with two performances in the States before leaving—the goal was to enable him to make it through the upcoming tour and then resume therapy upon his return.

Beginning with Investigative Touch, and knowing that a reactive protective response would need to be relieved first, I explored the way the humerus (the principal upper-arm bone) was sitting in the shoulder joint both while he was sitting up and lying down. The head of the humerus was jammed up with the rotator cuff muscles holding it fast into the glenoid/humeral socket, while keeping the scapulae held close in to the ribs by the serratus (anterior and posterior superior) and rhomboids. Simultaneously, the erector spinae was static in reactive response to the trauma from the fall, followed by overuse when he was conducting.

Switching to Engaged Touch, I had him lie face down, and then followed the contour of the outer ridge of the erector spinae (iliocostalis cervicus, longissimus thoracis, and ilio lumborum), using overlapping strokes from the bottom of the c-spine. I covered two or three vertebrae per stroke, working continuously down to the iliac crest. As this large group of muscles released their holding patterns, I then addressed the rotator cuff muscle group with similar strokes, using thumb pressure followed by a gentle peeling back of the serratus anterior and deltoid to access the triceps lateral and long head tendons. Here I applied Engaged Touch, using my thumb to work between release and pressure, gently but firmly, until I felt the release of the humerus from its position stuck in the socket. Then I addressed the rhomboids with similar strokes.

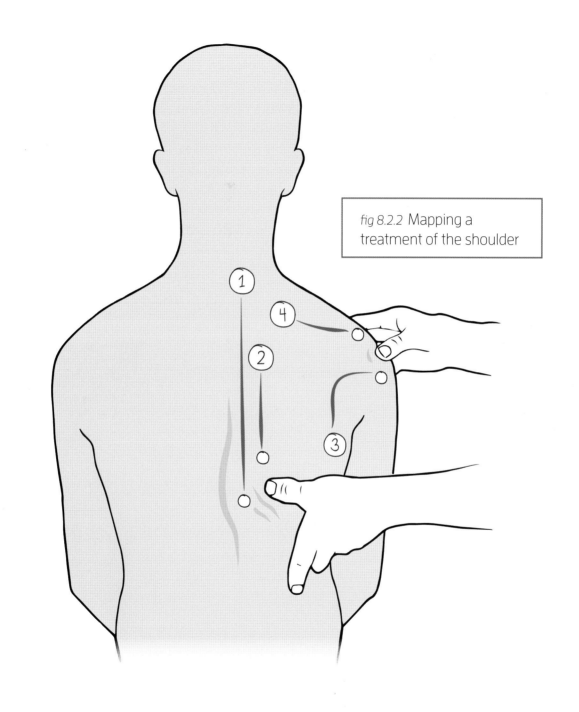

fig 8.2.2 Mapping a treatment of the shoulder

I chose my next step based on how much release had occurred and how much discomfort he was feeling. Because he was not overly reactive, I turned him onto his left side, then placed a pillow under his head and one between his knees. I placed a third one against his torso so I could drape the right arm over it, and with Investigative Touch, I took the right arm at the elbow and gently moved the arm and shoulder up, bringing the arm over and behind the head, stopping before it caused pain. This allowed me to judge how the front of the shoulder was restricting the normal movement of the arm through the shoulder joint.

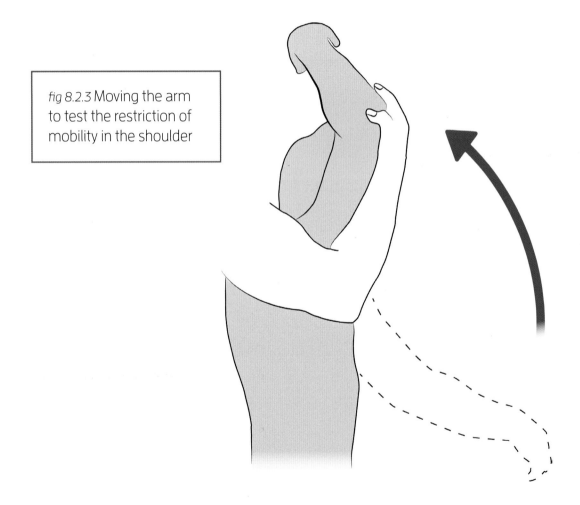

fig 8.2.3 Moving the arm to test the restriction of mobility in the shoulder

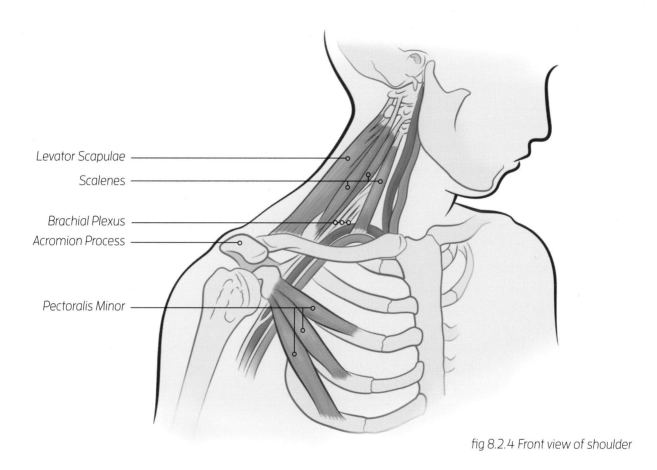

Levator Scapulae

Scalenes

Brachial Plexus

Acromion Process

Pectoralis Minor

fig 8.2.4 Front view of shoulder

Often the pectoralis major and minor are a bit contracted, as are the proximal and distal parts of the bicep muscle. Applying Engaged Touch to release the contracted tissues in these areas will usually complete the session, as it releases the pressure on the moving parts (including the nerves and blood vessels) and eases the symptoms. I followed up with another session the next day, and the maestro headed off on his international tour a couple of days later.

The shoulder is particularly tricky because the depth of the socket is shallow, making its stability and integrity dependent on the harmonious collaboration of bone, ligament, tendon, and muscle.

When analyzing shoulder pain, you have to consider the way the arm is moving in relation to the shoulder. Is the shoulder being held up primarily by the trapezius muscle and levator scapulae, or is it held down by the teres, serratus, and latissimus dorsi? Carefully observing the shoulder in action can help you determine where the imbalance lies.

Questions you might ask include: Is there restriction and/or pain when the subject raises the arm to the front, the side, or the back? Is there restriction and/or pain when the subject holds an object? Is there restriction and/or pain in rotation of the arm? The height to which the arm is raised determines which set of muscles hold the shoulder in place and which muscles move the arm. If the head of the humerus bone is not able to glide properly in the joint, it may inhibit the smooth movement of all the working parts, causing pain.

The most common mistake that therapists make when treating the shoulder is to work directly on the most painful area. This can actually cause more irritation while not addressing the root of the problem, which is the muscles that need to be released in order to allow normal function.

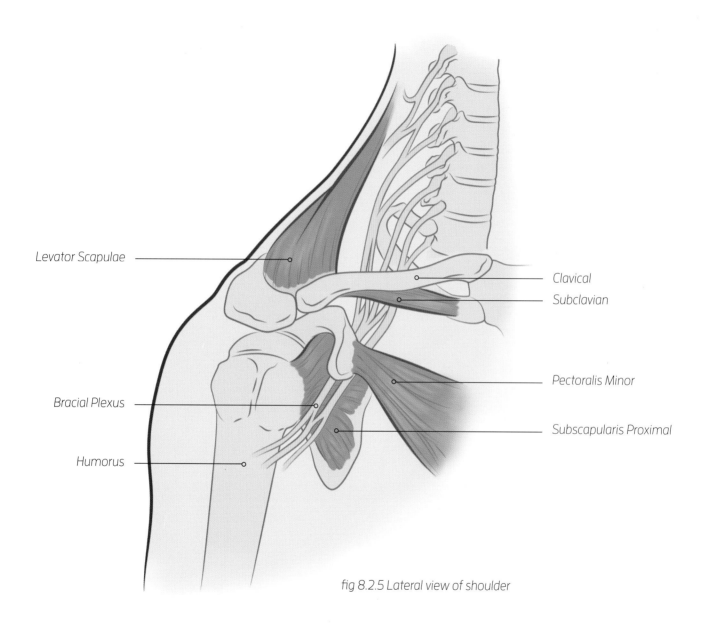

Levator Scapulae

Bracial Plexus

Humorus

Clavical

Subclavian

Pectoralis Minor

Subscapularis Proximal

fig 8.2.5 Lateral view of shoulder

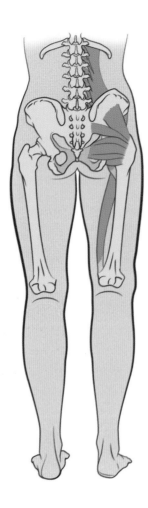
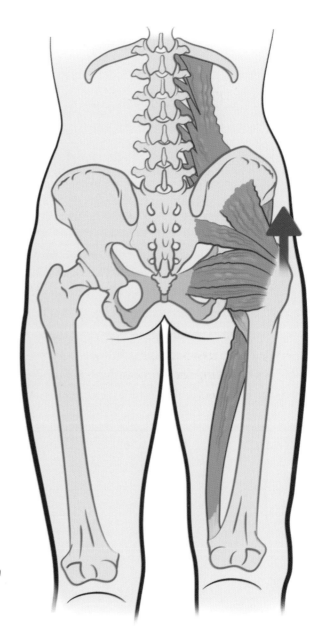

fig 8.3.1 Mapping irregularities and pain within the kinetic chair of the posterior view of the lower back and hip area. See appendix for anatomy detail

Lower Back

More and more people throughout the world are spending more and more time sitting at desks and work stations—and not surprisingly, therapists are treating more and more cases of the lower back pain that can result. And the problem is not just the pain itself; the pain often, in turn, makes it hard to concentrate, which results in less efficient work, which results in self-doubt and performance anxiety. Most injuries are similar—they create a chain-reaction, which means that solving for pain can have a ripple-effect that improves many other aspects of the subject's life.

Lower back pain develops like all repetitive stress injuries; tension accumulates gradually until what began as a slight stiffness becomes debilitating spasms in the muscles of the back and hips. Because many people sit for hours at a time, they overuse certain muscles; as those muscles get tired, they begin to slouch. Take the example of my editor. A literature professor, she lives on the east coast during the academic year, then moves to Paris for the summer to write and translate, all the while traveling as often as possible to the San Francisco Bay Area to visit her aging mother. All in all, she spends hours on end sitting—at a computer, on a plane, or at a table reading and writing. In this position, drooping shoulders compress the muscles of the lower back and hips, dropping the top of the pelvis back and loading more upper body weight and strain on the lumbar spine. This ends up limiting the space that the nerves have to pass through the hips to the legs; the restriction irritates the nerve tissues, tightening the muscles in these areas even more, which restricts the passage even more, and so on. I haven't treated her for this yet—she's on her way to see me, but is currently stuck in Logan airport, sitting at a sushi bar writing this sentence—but when she gets here, I'll have her lie face up with a supportive cushion under her knees to take the lumbar spine out of extension.

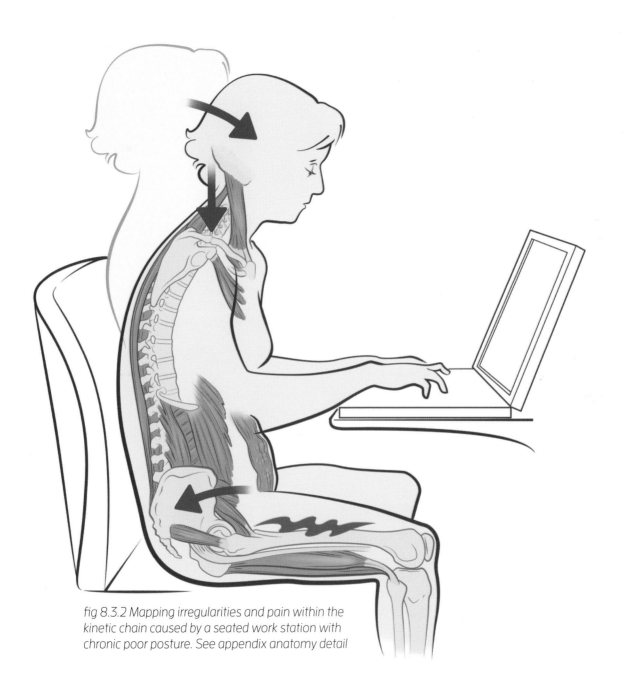

fig 8.3.2 Mapping irregularities and pain within the kinetic chain caused by a seated work station with chronic poor posture. See appendix anatomy detail

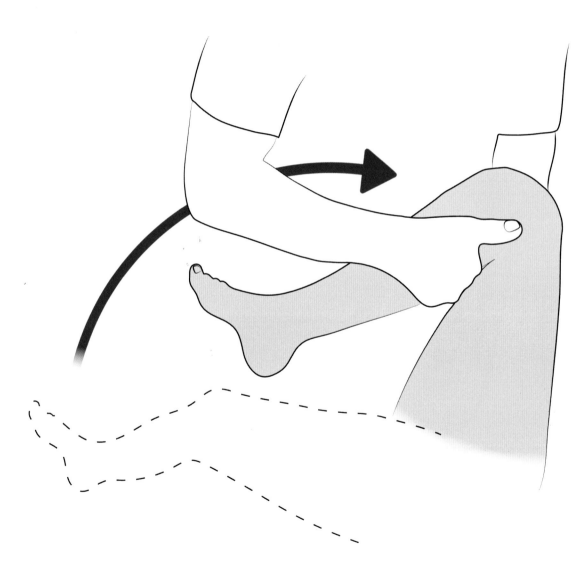

fig 8.3.3 Moving the leg to feel access areas within the mayo-fascial fabric

To relieve the tightness in and around the pelvis, begin by holding a knee with one hand while the other hand is placed on top of the iliac crest at the spot where the psoas, iliacus, and sartorius muscles come together. Lift the knee to gently flex the hip while applying Engaged Touch to the iliacus and the head of the sartorius, feeling for the subtle access areas within the mayo-fascial fabric. Press and semi-release while flexing and extending the hip from the knee as you maintain gentle firmness with Engaged Touch. Move the hand in contact with the pelvis muscles medially (to the left if you are working on the right side, to the right if you are working on the left side) until you sense the psoas under your thumb. Repeat this gentle movement of the hip, feeling for the release that indicates that the muscles within the kinetic chain have reset and returned to their natural state, relieving the nagging pain.

Next, address the back muscles (erector spinae group) and the quadratus lumborum, as explained above.

Often there is immediate relief, but if not, following up with one or two more sessions should be enough to give significant relief for this common condition.

In all cases, the therapist's touch is actually the extension of the subject's awareness of his or her own position in relation to the ideal, relaxed, released state. Daily routine, simply because it is routine, often distracts us from noticing how we're responding to stress—both positive and negative. And this leads to imbalance—not only physical, but also mental, emotional, and spiritual.

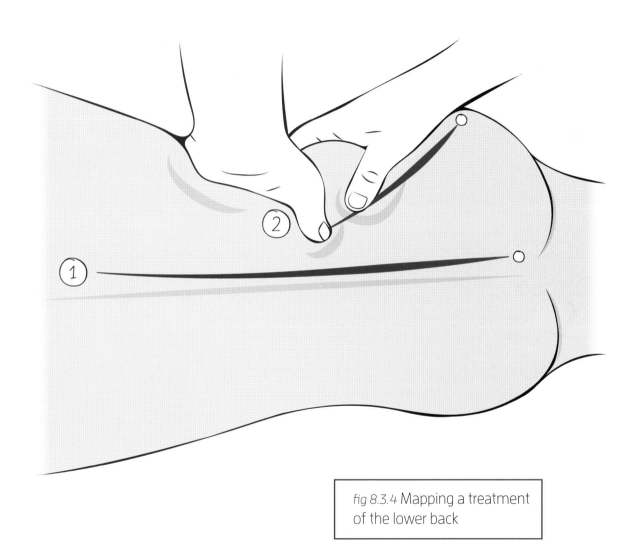

fig 8.3.4 Mapping a treatment of the lower back

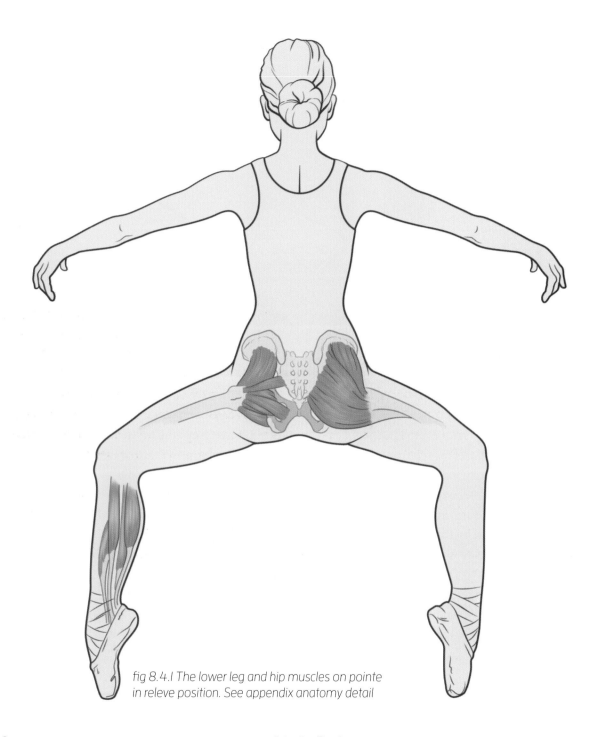

fig 8.4.1 The lower leg and hip muscles on pointe in releve position. See appendix anatomy detail

Intentive Touch

Lower Leg

`Several years ago, Tina LeBlanc, a principal dancer with the San Francisco Ballet, was preparing for an international tour when a pain in her calf became too much for her to bear, so she went to the ballet's medical staff for an evaluation and learned that the source of the pain was a small tear in the soleus muscle in her calf. The staff doctors suggested she take 6 to 8 weeks off to allow the muscle's fabric to knit back together and repair. But that international tour was only three weeks away. However, Tina was smart; she limited her preparation to the barre, worked only in flat ballet shoes (not pointe) for two weeks, and came to see me.

People who become truly excellent in their chosen lines of work—whether in athletics, entertainment, politics, or finance—often do so because they have the capacity to perform well under conditions of high stress. While this intensity is what sets them apart from the rest, it also creates the potential for illness and/or injury. They can overcome the physical and psychological pressures that come with their passion to achieve, but often only by ignoring the effects of the added stress until it manifests as acute pain and stops them in their tracks. In other words, the progression of stresses that leads to injury goes unnoticed until it is too late to keep it from affecting their exceptional performance.

When I examined Tina with Investigative Touch, I found that her entire calf was very tight with some of the gastrocnemius and soleus muscles in partial spasm. In order to continue dancing despite the pain, Tina had protected the injured area by using the intrinsic muscles within the foot to support the larger extrinsic flexors and extensors, which had become locked up because their fibers were frozen in their multifaceted contracted state. Because the contracted fibers didn't release, other muscles had to work harder to overcome their holding pattern, which caused imbalances that resulted in the partial tearing of the soleus muscle.

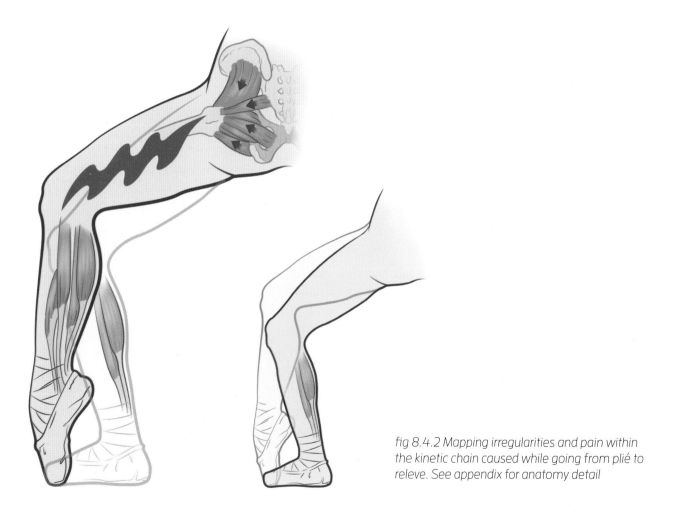

fig 8.4.2 Mapping irregularities and pain within the kinetic chain caused while going from plié to releve. See appendix for anatomy detail

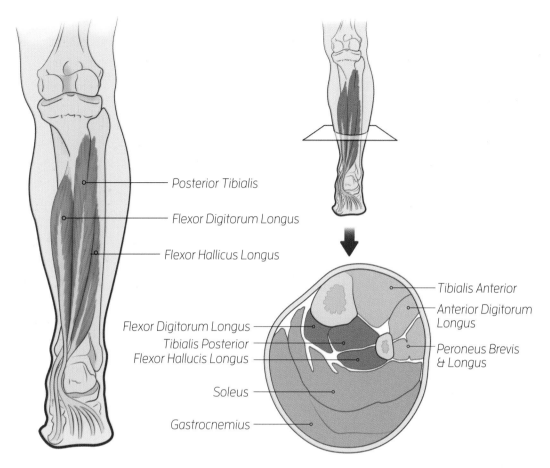

Posterior Tibialis

Flexor Digitorum Longus

Flexor Hallicus Longus

Tibialis Anterior

Anterior Digitorum Longus

Flexor Digitorum Longus

Tibialis Posterior

Flexor Hallucis Longus

Peroneus Brevis & Longus

Soleus

Gastrocnemius

fig 8.4.3 Muscle compartments of lower leg in posterior view and cross sections

Looking at the components of the lower leg shows how the muscles compensated and how the kinetic chain developed an irregularity. Tightness in the flexor digitorum and tibialis posterior keeps the foot from being able to glide under the leg so that to execute a proper plié, the plantar flexion needs the tibialis anterior to help pull the foot upward. This overuses the tibialis anterior, which in turn, causes its fibers to stay contracted and keeps the force of the body's action from releasing into the floor; instead, it stays in the contracted muscles, causing the fibers to tear.

Because every body is slightly different in size and shape, each acquires unique patterns of compensation to repair itself. But because there are only so many movements possible, the fix is close at hand. Interacting with the amazing machine that is the human body, Intentive Touch actually allows the body to fix itself by reducing the density of soft tissues with Engaged Touch so that the information for the self-regulating mechanisms is able to pass along the biological fascial fabric. In this case, it allowed the entire lower leg's muscle groups to release and return to a neutral resting state, similar to the way that a computer reboots itself after being shut off to avoid overheating.

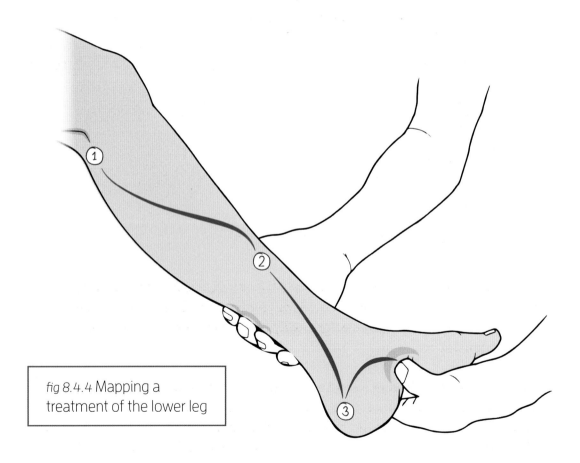

fig 8.4.4 Mapping a treatment of the lower leg

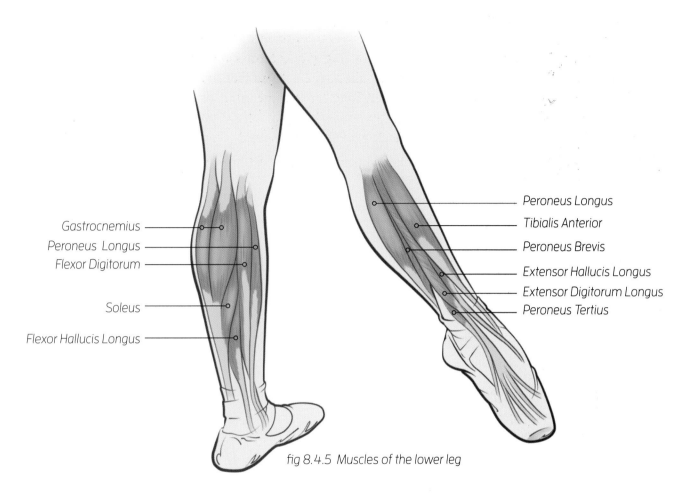

Gastrocnemius

Peroneus Longus

Flexor Digitorum

Soleus

Flexor Hallucis Longus

Peroneus Longus

Tibialis Anterior

Peroneus Brevis

Extensor Hallucis Longus

Extensor Digitorum Longus

Peroneus Tertius

fig 8.4.5 Muscles of the lower leg

In Tina's case, the combination of the inevitable overuse due to the intensity of a long ballet season and the demands of preparing for the lead role in the upcoming tour of Swan Lake had gradually caused her lower leg to evolve into this dysfunctional state.

LeBlanc danced the lead in Swan Lake by the end of the tour. Not only was she able to do that performance before the end of the eight weeks that she'd been advised to take off, but she did it with a much more informed and detailed picture of the complex physiological structures that made that performance possible.

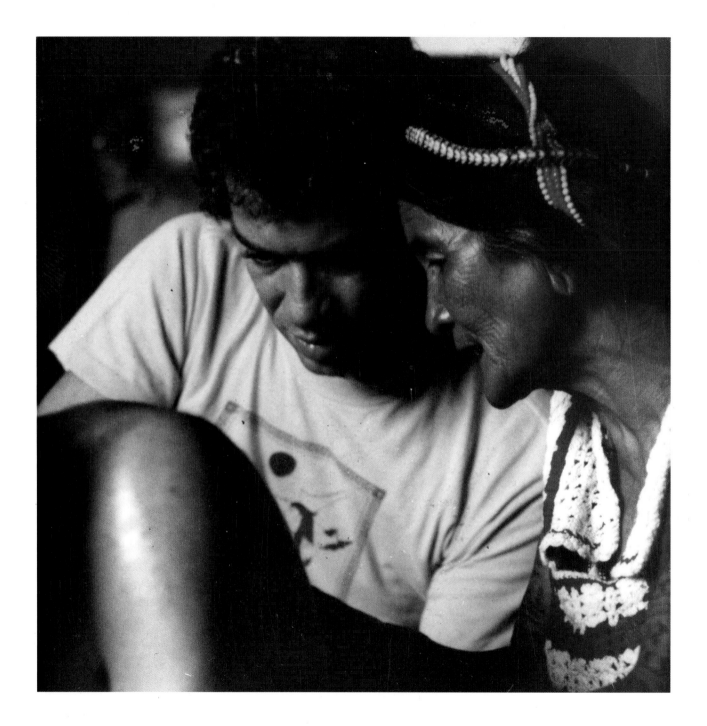

Intentive Touch

How I Learned the Healing Art of Hilot

Ina Facucad

A mile high, with a view that proves it, lies the city of Baguio, in the mountainous region of the Philippine island of Luzon. In a single sweep, the eye takes in a range of ridges and valleys in saturated blues and greens—the green of steep slopes, carefully terraced for growing rice, and the blues of a cloudless sky against distant hills, some several miles away. But I had not come for the scenery. It was 1979; I was 26 years old, and I had come seeking a way to help my 28-year-old brother, Gordon, who had been severely injured in a car accident the year before. In the face of his fractured spine and damaged spinal cord, traditional western medicine had little to offer, but Gordon had been involved in alternative and complementary medicine for years. At the time, he taught massage at the San Francisco School of Massage, where he was developing the curriculum for a therapeutic massage course. He spent the first four months after the accident in a hospital, researching all the possibilities for alternative treatment. He finally focused on the Philippines, which was getting a lot of press for its mysterious and miraculous healing arts. Meanwhile, I had shifted from budding rock-star to principal care-giver, bringing him home-cooked organic meals three times a day as well as boxes and boxes of research materials. As soon as Gordon could travel, we were on our way. And so, in December 1978, we found ourselves on a rickety bus winding up the side of an alarmingly rugged mountain many hours from the Manila International Airport.

Once we arrived, we did further research, which led us to the Filipina healer, Ina Facucad. That spring, I spent countless hours—day after day, for several months—in the Mountain Lodge Hotel, watching traditional healing at work on my paralyzed brother.

A small-framed woman in her 60s, Ina Facucad was tattooed from her hands to her elbows and dressed in the local traditional clothing, a wrap-around skirt woven with symbols of her tribe's mythologies. Her black, waist-length hair was tied up in strings of antique beads and snake vertebrae, and she kept a thin cigar tucked jauntily behind one ear. She handled Gordon with confident care, clearly a master at work in her prime.

And the results supported this impression. When we arrived, Gordon had been in constant pain since his accident, suffering violent leg spasms, terrible edema in his feet, recurring pressure sores on his feet, hips, and legs, and paralysis from the mid-nipple down. After three and a half months of Facucad's treatment, he had dramatically improved his sensations, eliminated the pressure sores, regained movement in his lower back muscles, regained sexual function, greatly reduced the edema in his feet, and was able to stand without braces between parallel bars.

One day Facucad arrived exhausted; she had just traveled 80 miles in a harrowing eight-hour bus journey from her home in a remote Bontoc village to Baguio City. She had come directly from the bus terminal in order to get the session started as soon as possible, and she was feeling the strain. So she asked me to help. As she spoke no English, and I spoke no Tagalog, we "talked" through hand gestures and facial expressions, but the communication seemed no less fluent for that.

But I was surprised that she had asked for my help—this had never happened before. As I followed her to the bed, she motioned for me to work on my brother's knee. I sat down beside her and began groping it clumsily. Ina Facucad took my hands and placed them on the top of Gordon's bent knee. I wanted to protest that I didn't know what to do but before I could, it was there – clearly – a sense of the contour of the upper leg meeting with the lower leg, with interstitial fluids and all the musculo-tendonous, neurovascular connective tissue attachments entering the joint capsule forming the knee. I could feel the imbalance of the muscle groups subtly pulsating with spasmodic waves of contraction. I could locate the balance points and calm the spastic waves allowing the leg to release the reactive patterning caused by the injury to his spinal cord. It was stunning! I pushed her hands away as if we had switched bodies. I felt like I was on auto-pilot and could just allow the process to happen. And it stayed with me, like a video clip that I could replay. Each time she worked, she would teach me to treat some new part of the body, and I could replay the lesson whenever I needed it.

In retrospect, I think my being in the Philippines, away from routine distractions, had created a suspension of time and a shift of purpose for me, and my hours of watching Ina Facucad had attuned me in ways that I wasn't conscious of at the time. A window of opportunity had opened, and I was fascinated. The fascination, in turn, created the discipline I needed in order to learn, and from that moment, I turned my attention to absorbing everything this wise tribal woman would share.

One of her first lessons was patience. Only through patience would the proper solutions reveal themselves. I spent the better part of the years between 1979 and 1985 with her. I worked mostly on Gordon, but once the very small community of people with spinal cord injuries heard of our travels and of Gordon's improvements, I was inundated with questions about how to get to see Ina Facucad. In the summer of 1979, two young men with spinal cord injuries made the trip to Baguio, and I worked beside Ina Facucad on my brother and his two mates. Over the next four years I worked both in the Philippines and in the United States on people with spinal cord injuries, including the case of a young man in San Diego, Bob White, who had suffered a broken neck in a motocross event and made a miraculous recovery.

Ina's full name was Alicia Facucad Fanged, and she was a master healer from a tribal community still practicing ancestor worship and animal sacrifice in the Cordillera Mountains of the northern Philippine island of Luzon. They lived by farming, raising rice by terracing the province's steep mountains. Ina had learned her healing skills from her mother, who had learned them from her mother, and so on, going back for many generations. She was also what they call Supok, a shaman. She had us call her Ina or Ina Facucad, as Ina means mother in her Bontoc dialect. A few years after we met her, she told me that before we had met, she had seen me in a dream carrying a paralyzed man. Clearly, I was meant to be there.

One of the invaluable lessons I learned was how to accept and be accepted by a fundamentally different world-view. Coming from the San Francisco Bay Area, where I had been a musician, playing guitar in rock groups, finding myself suddenly the protégé of a traditional shamanistic healer in a remote mountain community was nothing short of a shock. Gradually, I adjusted to the very slow pace of tribal village life and learned how to interpret and apply the unspoken concepts that Ina shared with me. She explained a fundamentally simple way to address the idiosyncrasies of the body:

First, conceptualize a basic map of the body; the body is made up of blood, bone, meat, and veins (urat and pennent). The meat is all the muscle, fat, tendon, and connective tissue. The term "blood" means not only blood itself, but also all other fluids, both interstitial and lymphatic.

The term "veins" here means not only the conduits from artery to capillary that carry basic blood, but all the tissue structures that carry all the various fluids throughout the body, as well the layers of tissues as they appear in cross section, and the energetic channels as understood by Chinese medicine.

The goal is to balance the meat on the bone, so that the blood will flow through the veins.

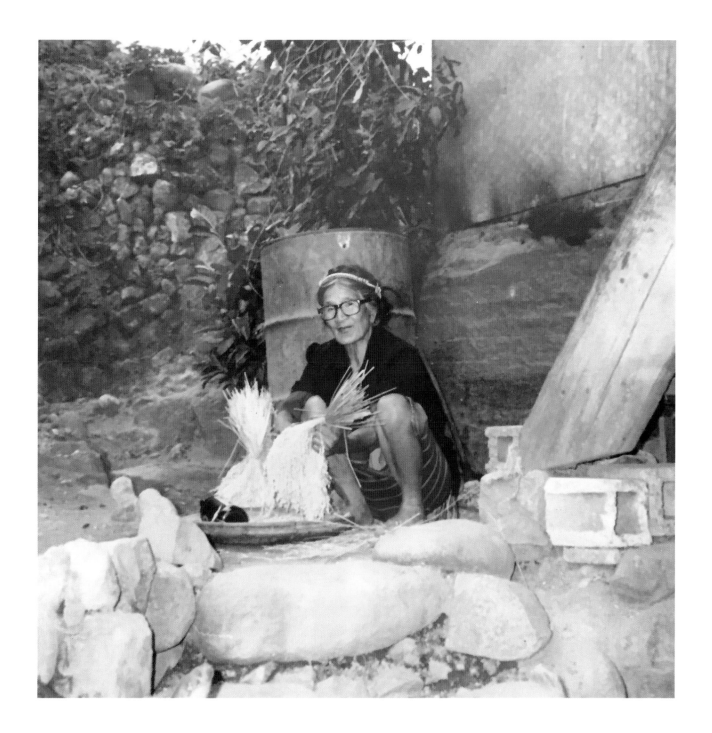

How I Learned the Healing Art of Hilot

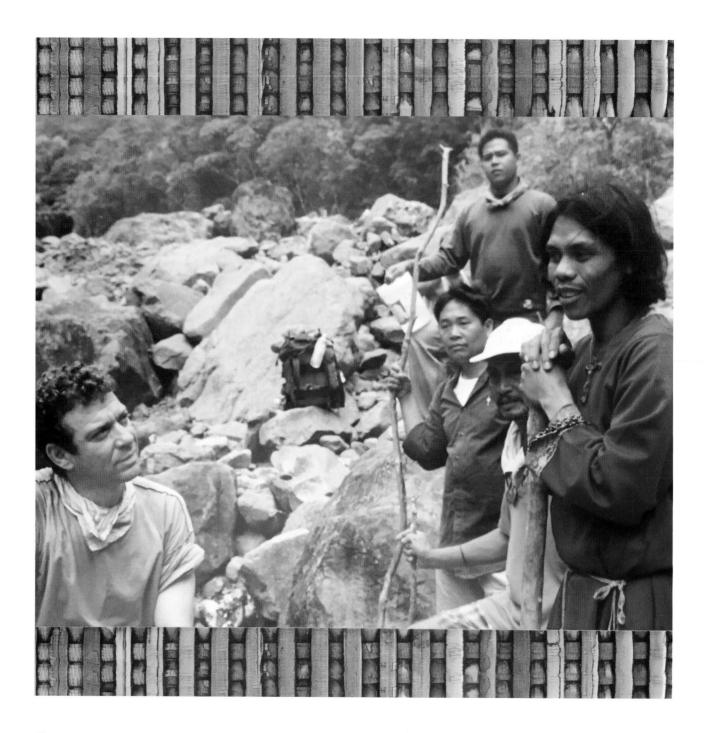

Intentive Touch

Other Healers

In 1985, after nearly five years of working intensively with Ina Facucad, I came back to the United States, but until her death in 2008, I returned frequently to visit and study with her. As the years went by, I also encountered other master healers who very generously shared their knowledge with me through hands-on teaching.

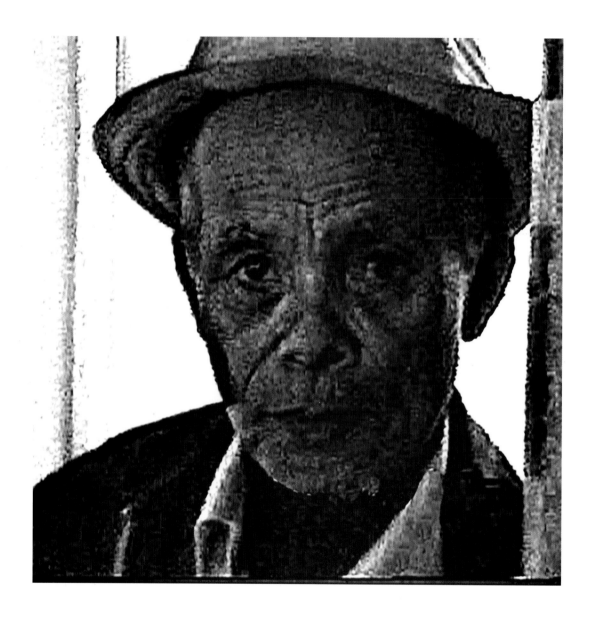

Intentive Touch

Anselmo Estacio

I met Anselmo in 1984 and worked with him from then until 1986. He was the gardener for a large estate in Baguio City, up the street from where we were living on Outlook Drive. When we met, he was 80 years old, and quite an interesting man. He came from a region called Naguilian, in the foothills below Baguio City, on the route to the South China Sea. He began each session with a silent prayer; then, after rubbing coconut oil on his fingertips, he would make the sign of the cross over the part of the subject's body that he was going to work on. His method was twofold. He always spoke (his English was quite good) of the need to balance hydraulic pressure. His method relied on applying touch to the connective tissue components at either end of the tendons that attach the muscle to the joint capsules. His touch was very light and, unlike Ina Facucad, he used very little coconut oil. He would spread his fingers wide and gently place his hands, fingertips only, ever so lightly, yet firmly, on the skin. This light touch was amazingly effective because of his sensitivity to the subtle changes beneath his fingertips. The results were remarkable, but initially, it was a difficult technique to copy. It was so different from Ina Facucad's that at first I didn't know what to do during sessions with my subjects, but I eventually learned to incorporate aspects of his practice, particularly his way of examining subjects, into what was increasingly becoming my own unique practice based on a hybrid of all I had learned.

Anselmo was also a master herbalist, using botanicals that he collected locally as well as in his native region. He blended the plants to make compresses, which he used to soften hardened and matted tissues and to treat burns and other injuries and illnesses.

Anselmo didn't have a "lineage" per se; instead, he was one of the many healers throughout the Philippines who have gotten most of their knowledge through dreams. In Anselmo's case, and perhaps because he was a devoted Catholic, the Virgin Mary appeared in his dreams and instructed him in healing practices. Most healers who learn from their dreams report that they come suddenly and concretely; in Anselmo's case, the knowledge came to him when he was already an adult.

Trining Urbano

Trining was the youngest of the healers that I studied with; I met her in 1990, when she was in her early fifties, and worked with her until 1994, when she died at the age of 56. A robust 4' 10" tall, she was strong as a water buffalo and always smiling. She came from the Bicol area of Luzon, which is known for, among other things, Mount Mayon, one of the earth's rare perfectly symmetrical active volcanoes. Trining had been trained by a master healer from the Bicol region whose learning was based in the sacred Mount Banahaw tradition. This tradition comes from the island of Luzon, south of Manila, and relies heavily upon the writings of the early 20th century mystic Sabino, particularly a book titled Karunungan ng Diyosby, which might be translated as God's Wisdom. A collection of mystic, mythical, and esoteric stories, it develops the idea of breath as life, based on the theory that everything in the universe has its own unique frequency, and that frequencies are the common denominator of all the elements that make up the material world. Frequencies can be used to effect change, and can be deployed by chanting a mantra, a spell, or an incantation. Even the frequencies particular to words or names can have strong effect. The Karunungan ng Diyosby and this practice—like the practices of all the healers I worked with—were developed in the Philippines before the arrival of western influences, when the mystical was an essential and seamlessly integrated aspect of daily life.

Trining, whose English was very strong, described her work as a form of magnetic healing rooted in an active battle between good and evil and played out in the unseen "vibrational realms." She used significant force in her hands-on work—she really pushed. Using superficial-looking, quick, circular movements that followed the course of energy streams (similar to those used in Chinese medicine), she achieved a deep penetration. As she worked, she would often perspire, and heat radiated around her body and came off her hands. Along with her forceful touch, she also called upon the assistance of spirit helpers through oration, an incantatory practice in which words and phrases are silently repeated in a language that blends the native tongue with a pseudo-Latin.

Intentive Touch

As she silently chanted, Trining would follow the pathways of the neurovascular bundles and energy channels, at times using forceful strokes, and at times, gentle ones, all with the intention of clearing blocked energy.

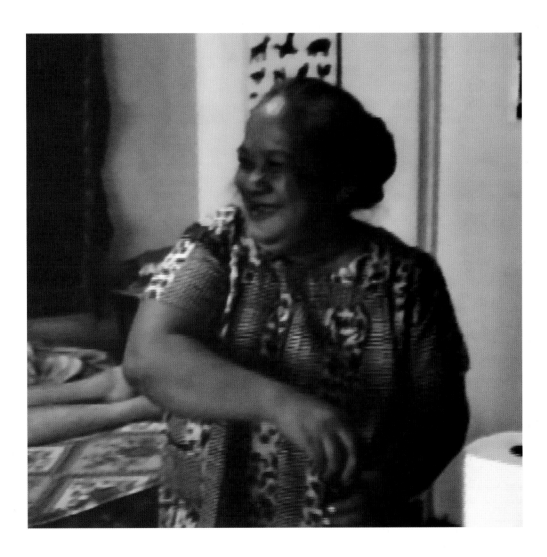

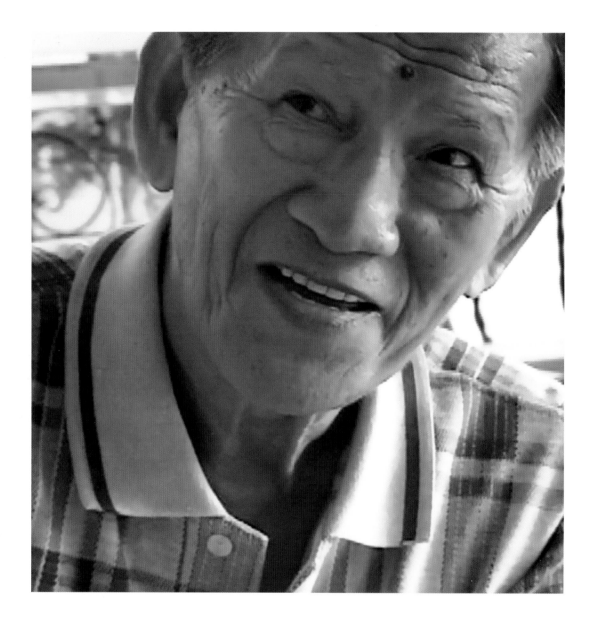

Intentive Touch

Anghel Caasi

I began working with Anghel Caasi in 1998, when he was a youthful 75 years old. He had been practicing for decades, using a traditional healing method from his hometown in Pangasinan, north of Manila, just before the foothills leading to Baguio. His method was strikingly different from all the others I had encountered, in that he first used friction, rubbing across the muscle fibers to begin to melt down their resistant tension, and then switched to an acupressure-type directed touch. Sometimes he would place one hand on a part of the body and the other over his head, like an antenna, as if it were receiving signals from above. He blended these local techniques with traditional Chinese medicine (TCM) and its mapping of affective points throughout the body. He would apply the focused touch to various points and then note the subject's responses, using different touches for an acupuncture point, a reflex point, or a tight muscle or tendon. Anghel was also different in that he was a professor of anatomy and physiology at the University of the Philippines, and could explain what he was doing both in western and eastern terms, and in fluent English.

Ultimately, I realized that there are many approaches and that they all can be used successfully to resolve any given problem. Not only does one method not invalidate the others, but in fact they often augment each other in a synergistic way. Thus, based on their common fundamental principles, I have slowly fused these diverse practices into a synthesis of all that I learned, further augmenting it with concepts and fundamentals from western medicine, where appropriate. This multi-perspective approach is particularly flexible and can be easily adapted to address any subject's specific problems.

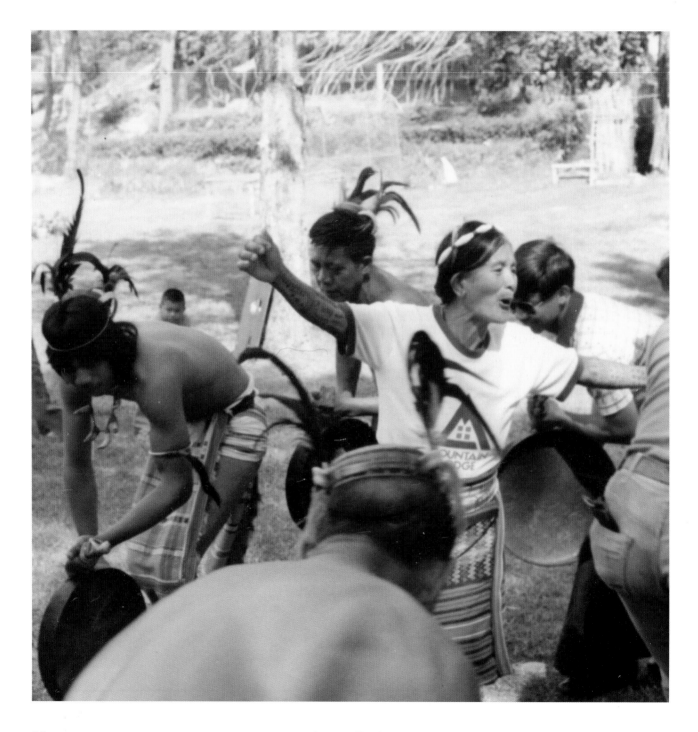

Intentive Touch

The Role of the Spiritual

Among the principles common to these diverse practices is a belief that the human experience, including its illnesses and injuries, is always a blend of the physical, mental, emotional, and spiritual aspects of a person's life, and each aspect affects all the others. In the pre-western culture of the Philippines, virtually everyone believed in the spirit world, and each area had its particular spirits. Some of these spirits were earth spirits, affecting natural phenomena, while others helped or hindered animals, including humans. When the Spanish occupied the Philippines in the late 16th century, they brought Christianity, and, as happened in many other parts of the world, traditional animistic spiritual beliefs and rituals became incorporated into Christian symbols and ideas. However, many regions of the Philippines were too remote to ever be touched by Christianity, and in such places, indigenous tribal traditions remained intact, and their relationship with the spirit world is unchanged. Today, each region of the 7000-island archipelago has its own type of spirituality. Whenever we connected with and worked with a healer, he or she would insist on sharing the local spiritual beliefs and knowledge with me, and I quickly came to understand that they all saw these spiritual beliefs as having a direct and important impact on the work itself. Despite the differences in details, I also quickly grasped that their spiritual beliefs, like my own, were all based in the common principle of love exercised through attention and compassion. It is important to keep a feeling of oneness with your subject and to remain always mindful of the intent to do good. The healer is the channeling mechanism for the world's positive energy, and keeping your mind clear, compassionate, and optimistic is key to keeping the channels between you and your subject clear and flowing smoothly.

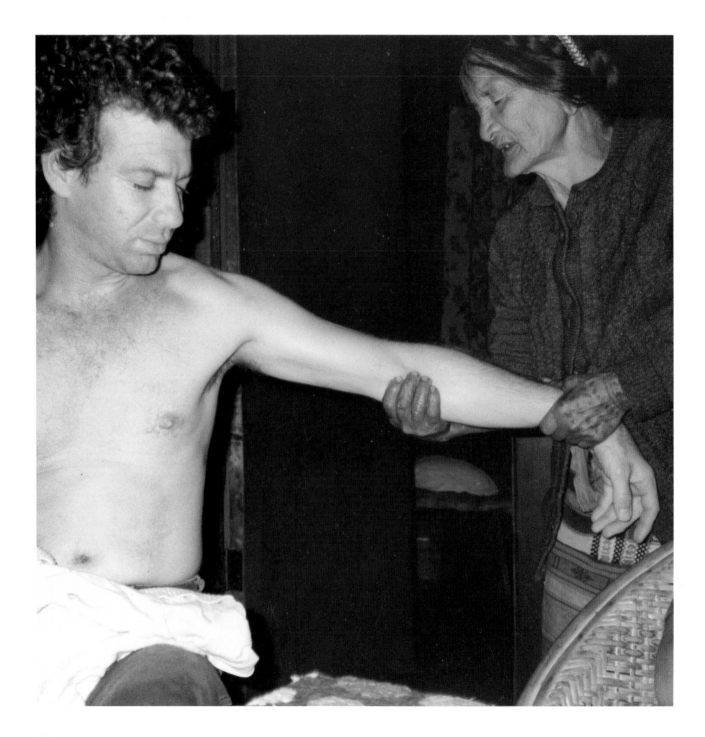

Intentive Touch

Self Awareness - Protection - Permission

All traditions view a human life as an interdependent blend of the physical, mental, emotional, and spiritual forces. And just as those aspects all influence each other within a given person, they also influence others, particularly people in close association. You, will be in close association with people facing some degree of challenge with one or more of these forces, and you need to be aware of conflictual energy, which can deplete your own.

Thinking optimistically, these situations create opportunities to reflect on our own personal conflicts. And in helping others we can find solutions for ourselves as well. Initially, I felt a need for protection from these negative forces, but as time passed, and interactions brought up similar issues, I found that accepting yourself creates a generous environment and allows you to feel good and to heal. Protection therefore is a by-product. But in my early years I depleted my life force easily and often and wasn't sure how to find my way.

Trining was the first healer who made sure I actively addressed this issue, discussing various ways that healers can protect themselves. Later I realized that Ina Facucad had also been trying to explain this necessity to me when she told me to "kill a chicken." It just didn't make sense to me at the time, but gradually I came to understand that, in her tradition, which includes animal sacrifice, the spirit of the chicken appeases other unseen but controlling spirits. It's like an insurance policy against the ills of many stresses—in my case, the pains and exhaustion a healer is in danger of absorbing from the people he routinely works on.

While Facucad's solution may seem dramatic to someone in the western world today, it acknowledges the very real psychic and physical costs that the healer incurs, and it foregrounds the role that belief, or mental intentionality, plays in alleviating their negative effects.

Though they may call it by different names, all the healers I worked with recognized this drain, even—if it's not putting it too strongly—this danger. Their ways of addressing it differed, depending upon their spiritual beliefs and their traditions, but all their methods had common underlying principles.

One is the need for self-awareness. Before you can help anyone effectively, you must know how to assess yourself and to establish boundaries for yourself. Learning to conserve energy by observing how you manage your energy throughout your daily routine is fundamental to helping others.

To maintain your own energy and to nourish yourself in general, be aware that the healing source is accessed through the subtle energies that reveal themselves when the mind is quieted and we feel at ease and confident. There are as many ways to attain this state, including well-known disciplines such as meditation, prayer, yoga, Tai Chi, and Chi Gong.

Each of us has our own core beliefs, which determine our path in life. If your path leads you to try to help relieve the suffering around you, then a method for conserving your energy will reveal itself to you. The disciplines listed above are often successful approaches.

Love, Compassion, and Healing

I've developed a particular meditation that I've found to be very successful for protecting my life force. It's based on Trining's practice of repeating charged words, modified by something I heard at a Chi Gong meditation class, in which the Chi Gong master, Min Tong Gu, suggested that before beginning the exercises, we should respectfully project our intention for love, compassion, and healing.

The meditation itself is very simple: either sitting, standing, or lying down, project your intention for love, compassion, and healing in all six directions:

1. Out the front of your body
2. Out the back of your body
3. Out the left side of your body
4. Out the right side of your body
5. Out the top of your head
6. Out the bottom of your feet

This exercise is based on the notion that "like attracts like" and assumes that what we project will come back to us.

Meditation Example

In this case, it's love, compassion, and healing that will be attracted back from all six directions, creating a field of like energy to draw from and allowing you to preserve your own life force and be revitalized in the process.

Once you are comfortable in the practice, you can add the actual directions in space.

1. Front=East
2. Back=West
3. Left=North
4. Right=South
5. Top=Above
6. Bottom=Below

This is only one example, and if it doesn't appeal to you, don't use it, but some form of such protection is important, so do find and use something that works for you.

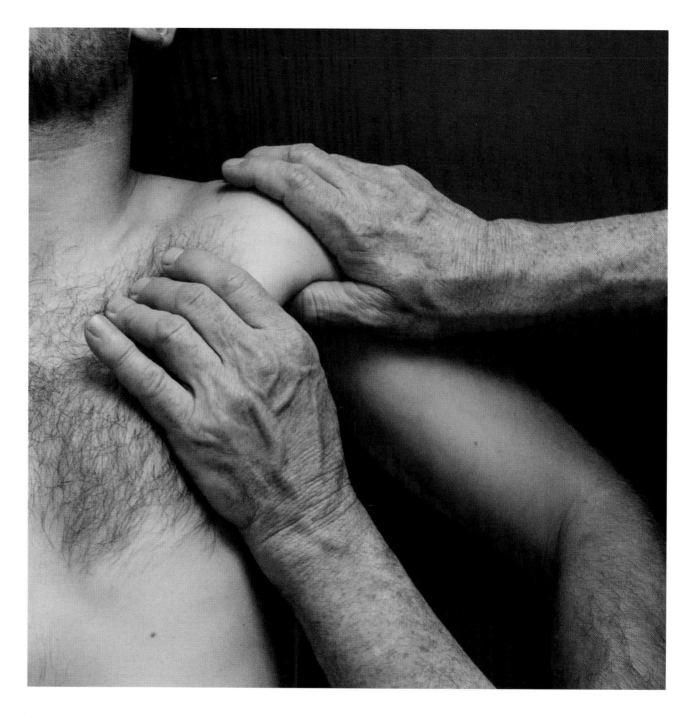

Intentive Touch

Concepts and Underlying Principles

- The body is an amazing machine, built of interactive layers of self-regulating mechanisms. It is designed to repair itself from all the things that happen to it throughout our lives. When not in balance, illness, pain, and disability occur.
- With the healing arts, the practitioner is not actually healing the body as much as he or she is finding ways to allow the body to heal itself.
- Keeping this in mind makes it easier to build and maintain the confidence necessary to use intuition and skills to help people to ease their pains and suffering.
- Allowing the body to return to balance is easier to achieve than you think.
- Intentive Touch allows the body to resume its self-regulation.
- Be patient and observe.
- Remember that there always are more layers revealing solutions, if you are open to the possibilities.

Intentive Touch is not an alternative therapy, but is a complimentary therapy, part of a community of practices that allow health care practitioners to interact together. These practitioners include physicians, physical therapists, nurses, all body workers, and other health care givers. Consulting such people and taking advantage of their considerable knowledge and experience can be extremely helpful to soft tissue therapists. Develop relationships with other health care workers in your community and refer to them whenever you have even the slightest doubt about a condition. This not only increases your knowledge, but also strengthens communication and builds community.

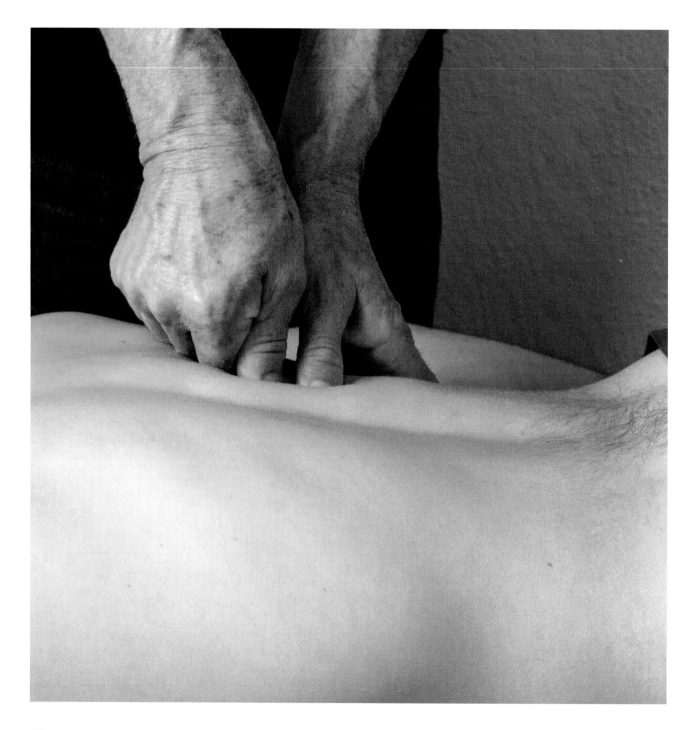

Intentive Touch

Appendix

Detailed Anatomy References

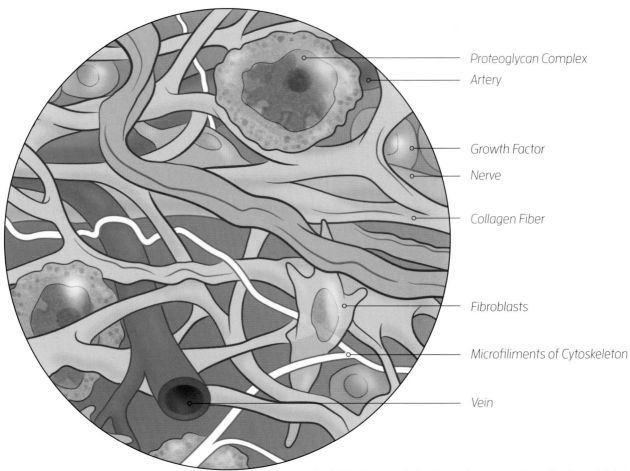

Proteoglycan Complex

Artery

Growth Factor

Nerve

Collagen Fiber

Fibroblasts

Microfiliments of Cytoskeleton

Vein

fig 3.2.1 – Extra Cellular Matrix / zooming into the fascial fabric

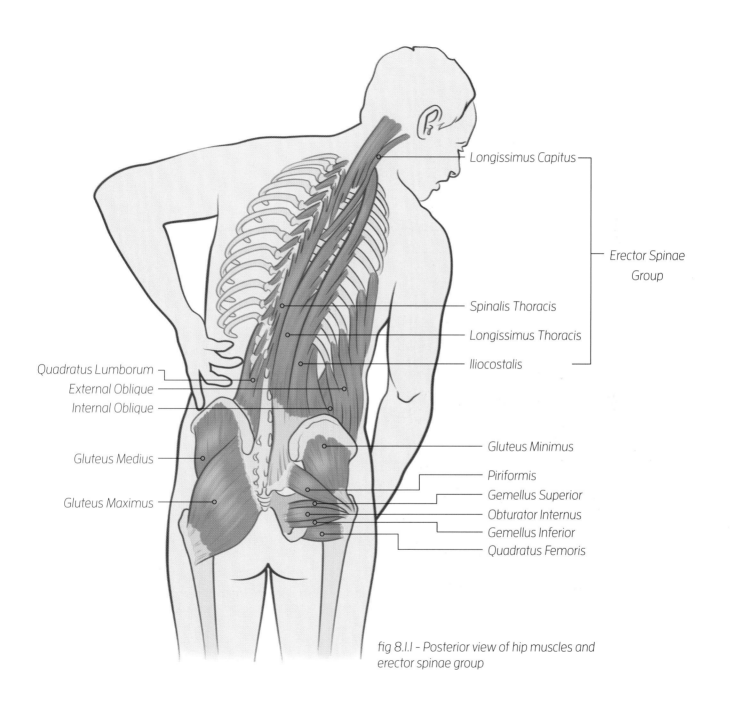

Longissimus Capitus

Erector Spinae
Group

Spinalis Thoracis

Longissimus Thoracis

Iliocostalis

Quadratus Lumborum

External Oblique

Internal Oblique

Gluteus Minimus

Piriformis

Gemellus Superior

Obturator Internus

Gemellus Inferior

Quadratus Femoris

Gluteus Medius

Gluteus Maximus

fig 8.1.1 - Posterior view of hip muscles and
erector spinae group

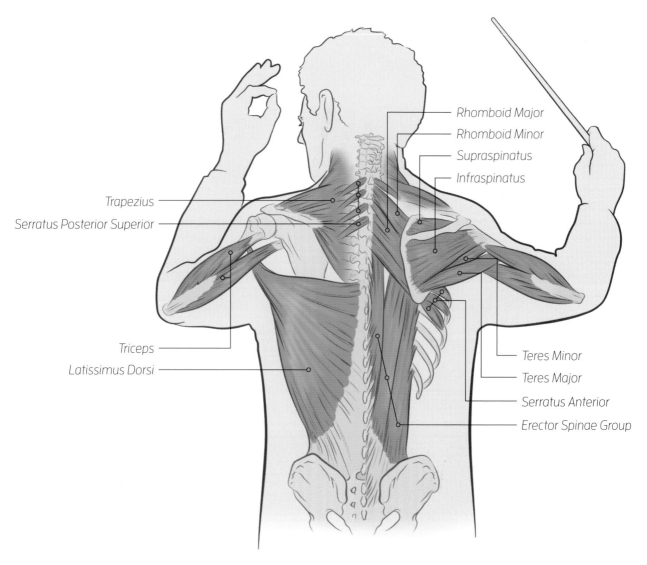

Rhomboid Major

Rhomboid Minor

Supraspinatus

Infraspinatus

Trapezius

Serratus Posterior Superior

Triceps

Latissimus Dorsi

Teres Minor

Teres Major

Serratus Anterior

Erector Spinae Group

fig 8.2.1 - Posterior view of back muscles

Intentive Touch

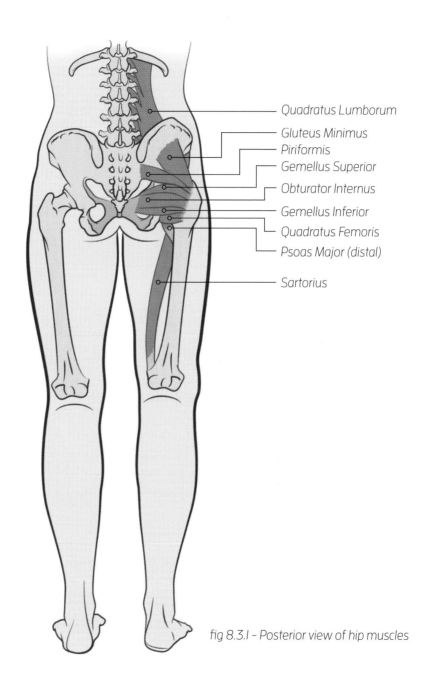

Quadratus Lumborum

Gluteus Minimus

Piriformis

Gemellus Superior

Obturator Internus

Gemellus Inferior

Quadratus Femoris

Psoas Major (distal)

Sartorius

fig 8.3.1 - Posterior view of hip muscles

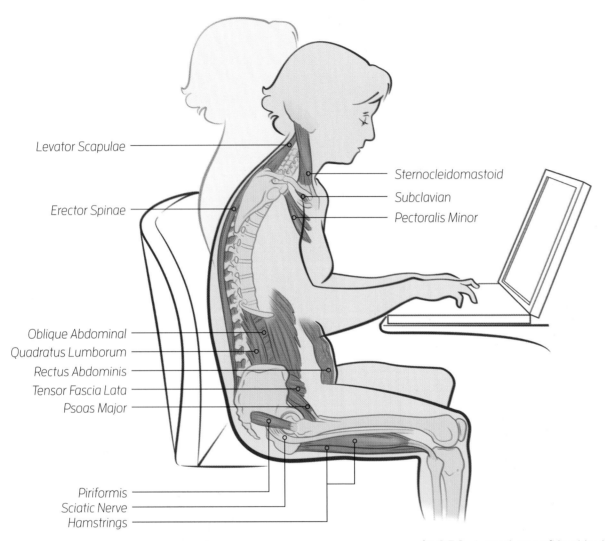

Levator Scapulae

Erector Spinae

Sternocleidomastoid

Subclavian

Pectoralis Minor

Oblique Abdominal

Quadratus Lumborum

Rectus Abdominis

Tensor Fascia Lata

Psoas Major

Piriformis

Sciatic Nerve

Hamstrings

fig 8.3.2 - Lateral view of shoulder, back, abdominal, hip, and leg muscles

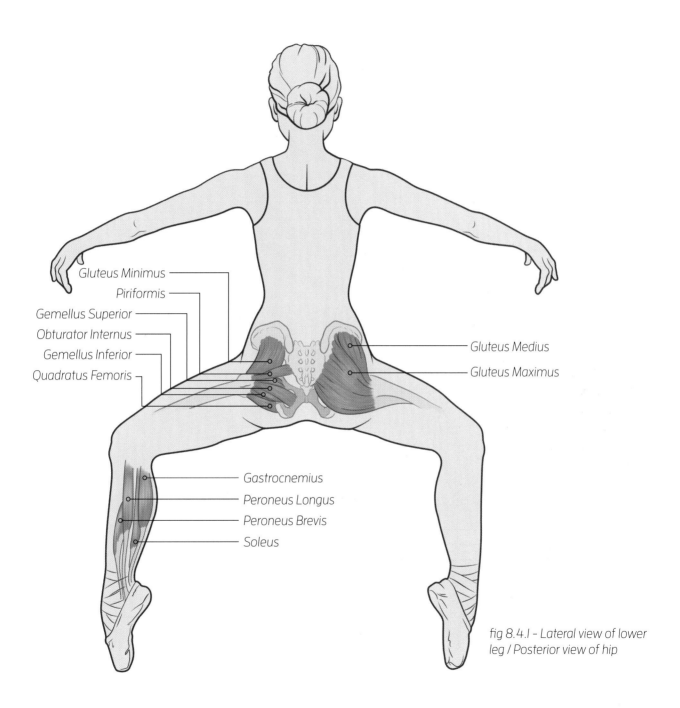

Gluteus Minimus

Piriformis

Gemellus Superior

Obturator Internus

Gemellus Inferior

Quadratus Femoris

Gluteus Medius

Gluteus Maximus

Gastrocnemius

Peroneus Longus

Peroneus Brevis

Soleus

fig 8.4.1 - Lateral view of lower leg / Posterior view of hip

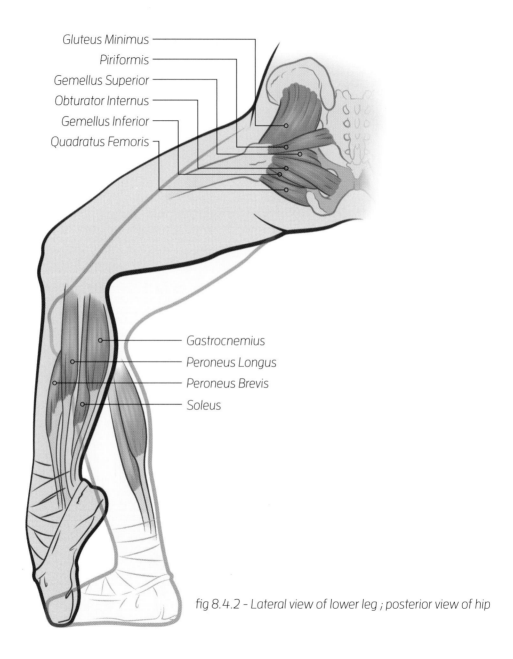

Gluteus Minimus

Piriformis

Gemellus Superior

Obturator Internus

Gemellus Inferior

Quadratus Femoris

Gastrocnemius

Peroneus Longus

Peroneus Brevis

Soleus

fig 8.4.2 - Lateral view of lower leg ; posterior view of hip

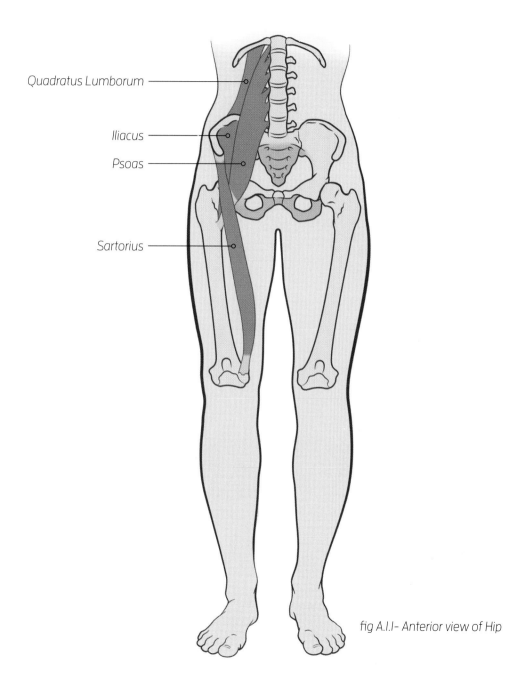

Quadratus Lumborum

Iliacus

Psoas

Sartorius

fig A.I.I- Anterior view of Hip

Primary Branches of the Cardiovascular System and Acupuncture Channels

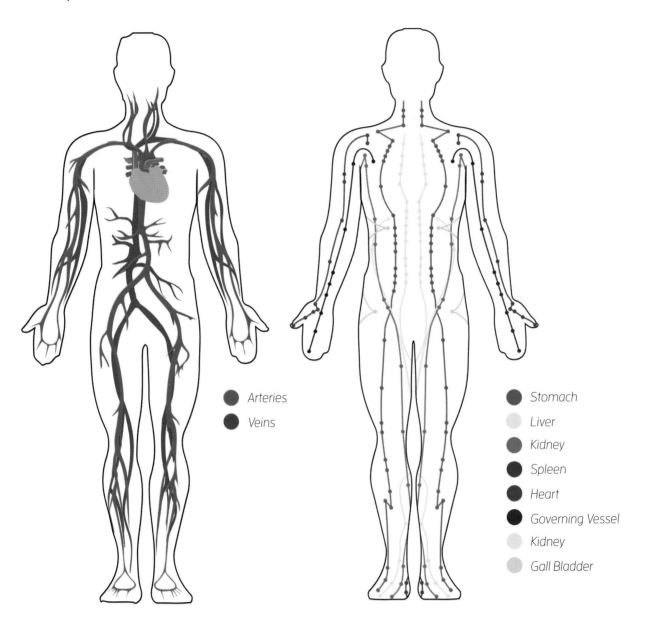

Arteries

Veins

Stomach

Liver

Kidney

Spleen

Heart

Governing Vessel

Kidney

Gall Bladder

Intentive Touch

Index

A

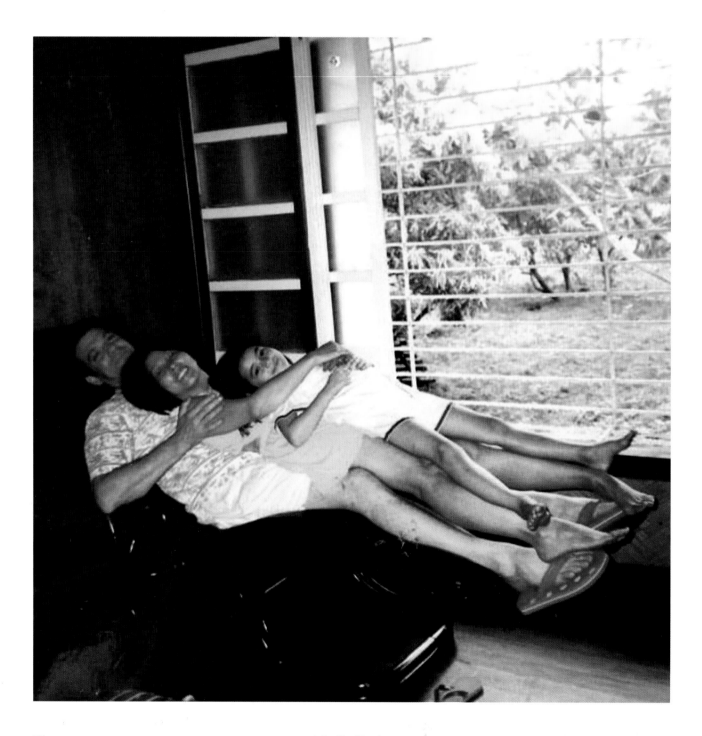

Intentive Touch

Dedications

To my wife Isabel, and daughter Willi, whose loving support made it possible for me to do this.

To my parents who gave me the opportunity to be grateful and happy to be alive.

Acknowledgements

In the spirit of community, there are many I gratefully acknowledge in my journey:

Gordon Cohen

Anne Cohen

Bo Razon

Javy Singh

Carmir Singh

Bong Cawed

Dick Cawed

Ina Facucad

The Fanged Family

Anselmo Estacio

Nanay Trining Urbano

Jack Urbano

Anghel Caasi

Matthew Brill

Danny Glover

Gerry Gerena

Egay Navarro

Tim Badger

Slate Werner

Fran Milner

Anne Hamersky

Laura Lichterman

Virgil Apostol

Mark Morris

Michael Tilson Thomas

Dr Paul Handleman

Dr. Paul Rossman

Tyler Bronstein

Steven Morse

George Rosenfeld

Marty Tibor

A special thanks to Cole Swensen, professor of literature at Brown University, for editing and Willi Cohen for book design and editorial contributions.

Footnotes

[1] *"Tenets of Osteopathic Medicine." Tenets of Osteopathic Medicine. N.p., n.d. Web. June 2015.*

[2] *"Fascia and Extra-Cellular Matrix - Stability and Movement." Anatomy Trains. N.p., n.d. Web. May 2015.*

[3] *"Fascia and Extra-Cellular Matrix - Stability and Movement." Anatomy Trains. N.p., n.d. Web. May 2015.*

[4] *Lichterman, Laura. Introduction to Hilot. Rep. Holistic Health Institute. n.p., 2012. Print.*

[5] *"Intrathecal." TheFreeDictionary.com. The Gale Group, Inc., 2008. Web. 08 June 2016.*

[6] *Korr, Irvin M. "Proprioceptors and Somatic Dysfunction, 1975." The Collected Papers of Irvin M Korr (1997): n. pag. Amer Academy of Osteopathy.*

[7] *Lichterman, Laura. Introduction to Hilot. Rep. Holistic Health Institute. n.p., 2012. Print.*

[8] *Apostol, Virgil Mayor. Way of the Ancient Healer: Sacred Teachings from the Philippine Ancestral Traditions. Berkeley, CA: North Atlantic, 2010. Print.*

[9] *Facucad Fanged, Ina. "Hilot." Philippines, Bontoc. 1980. Speech. Translated by Rhamond Kayang*

[10] *O'Connor, John, and Dan Bensky. Acupuncture: A Comprehensive Text. Chicago: Eastland, 1981. Print. Pages 9-10*

[11] *Ronell. "Fascia Magnified 25x (Subtitled)." YouTube. YouTube, 2013. Web. 12 Feb. 2014*

[12] *Biewener, Andrew A. "Muscles and Skeletons: The Building Blocks of Animal Movement." Animal Locomotion. Oxford: Oxford UP, 2003. N. pag. Print.*